26 Inservices for Activity Departments

Haley Burress

Idyll Arbor, Inc.
39129 264th Ave SE, Enumclaw, WA 98022 (360) 825-7797

Idyll Arbor, Inc. Editor: Thomas M. Blaschko
Cover design: Thomas M. Blaschko
Photo credit: © Nyul | Dreamstime.com

© Copyright 2016, Haley Burress.

All rights reserved. Forms may be copied for use in inservices. Idyll Arbor also grants the owner of this book the right to copy the stories from *The Enduring Human Spirit* used as part of inservices 24 and 25. No other part of this book may be reproduced, stored in a retrieval system, or transcribed, in any form or by any means — electronic, mechanical, photocopying, recording, web site, or otherwise — without the prior written permission of the publisher.

To the best of our knowledge, the information and recommendations of this book reflect currently accepted practice. Nevertheless, they cannot be considered absolute and universal. Guidelines suggested by federal law are subject to change as the laws and interpretations do. Recommendations for a particular client must be considered in light of the client's needs and condition. The authors and publisher disclaim responsibility for any adverse effects resulting directly or indirectly from suggested management practice or therapy technique, from any undetected errors, or from the reader's misunderstanding of the text.

ISBN 9781611580426

Contents

How to Use This Resource

Training staff is an important part of an Activity Director's job. Depending on the state that you work in, regulations suggest activity staff training of 10 or more hours per year. With paperwork, planning, and resident care, it can be difficult to schedule regular inservices. Finding topics and preparing materials takes time, too. This resource can be your guide for high quality training opportunities for your staff. Some of these inservices can be shared other departments in your community.

There are 26 lessons in this resource, including a list of nontraditional training ideas for you to use. Each of the lessons includes a training sign-in sheet already filled out with the content and goal of the session. If your community does not have a sign-in template, simply copy the sheet at the end of the lesson, fill in the blanks, and have participants sign in. Then give the sheet and any handouts to human resources for filing.

Each inservice has an overview at the beginning of the chapter. The overview includes:

Topics: A summary of what is covered in the inservice.

Who to Invite: Suggestions about other people to invite to the inservice. You may wish to invite only activity staff to your inservices. However, I encourage you to ask other staff to attend. Interdepartmental cooperation can be increased with increased understanding of each others' jobs.

Time: Estimated time for the inservice. Most of the inservices will take 30-60 minutes. The lecture parts are generally quite short. Most of the learning is done during activities and discussions. In setting the timing of the inservices, I assume each activity or discussion will take about five minutes.

Supplies: Material required for the inservice, including handouts.

Co-presenters: Some inservices will help explain how to work with another department. It will be helpful if representatives of both departments present information. Members of both departments can attend the inservice together to share ideas and concerns.

Review Material: Information that you might need to review or prepare in advance. A day or two before the scheduled training, take some time to go over the latest community, state-specific, or federal information.

Content Reminders: Brief reminders of specific content areas to include.

After the overview is the inservice itself. Each includes information, best practices, and ideas. It is my hope that you use the information as an outline for your presentation. Often you can present it pretty much as it is written. Other times the differences in each state, each community, and each department will require you to do some adaptation of the information you discuss.

There are multiple activities and discussion breaks in each lesson. During that time your staff and other attendees can try out ideas and share their community-specific issues or experiences. You should feel free to add your own experiences as well! In a collaborative environment, the experiences of all the members of the class can provide valuable ideas for everyone. Your staff look up to you and learn from your experiences, and you should learn from the experiences of your staff and other members of the healthcare team.

Note that most of the activities can be read to the group more or less as they are written. Note that some activities start with the word "process." For those, follow the process described as you lead the activity.

Consider scheduling inservices at least once a month. The more consistent you can be, the better. For example, always meet on the third Wednesday of the month at 2 p.m. Your inservice time should be all about learning. If you want to add a staff meeting for announcements, initiatives, etc., you can do that at the beginning or end of the inservice content. When members of other departments attend, don't take up their time with your department's work.

It is my hope that you will use these inservices to train your staff and make your department better. The end goal should be improved service for residents. If some of these inservices point out weaknesses in your department, embrace them and improve them. Use this chance to learn about best practices together as a team and then brainstorm how you can work together to make your program better. I suggest ending each inservice by developing one to three changes that you can make to your program over the next month, based on information that you learned.

Have fun learning together!

1.
Excitement is Contagious!

The importance of approach and attitude during invitation and facilitation of groups.

Topics
How to get the attention, and keep the attention, of residents in a group setting.
How to motivate residents to attend programs.
How to encourage residents to get involved in a group activity.

Who to Invite
Activity staff, CNA staff, caregiver staff, volunteers who lead groups.

Time
50-60 minutes.

Supplies
Inservice sign-in sheet.
Bingo cards and Bingo chips.

Co-presenters
CNA supervisor, volunteer supervisor.

Content Reminders
Remember to add your own personal experience and encourage sharing.

Attitude is everything. We've heard that saying before, and it certainly is accurate. Sometimes, we don't realize how much influence we have on a group or even on a person. However, when you're working with seniors, it is important to realize the impact that you have on your audience. Your attitude going into an interaction can drastically increase or decrease the number of participants in your program and how long residents stay. It can affect the mood of your group, too. No matter how you look at it, your attitude is important!

Activity

Let's try it out. Split into pairs. Person #1, tell your partner that it is time to go to gardening group … and don't be excited about it. All I want you to say is, "It's time for gardening group." Be sure to not look your partner in the eyes, and act a bit of a "Debbie Downer" when you say it. Person #2, did you really want to go to gardening group? Let's share some of your reactions.

When you approach residents, whether to simply start a conversation or to invite them to a group, your body language and voice are important. Bad days happen to all of us, but if we let it show to the residents, it can lead to decreased participation. Here's an example: You are having a bad day. You really don't like gardening group in the first place. You can't believe that your director wants you to lead gardening group *again.*

If all of that is going on, you might let it show in your attitude when you invite Susie Resident to the group. Then Susie is probably not going to want to come and plant flowers with you.

In a similar line, if you're having a busy day and know that you have to lead the 2 p.m. gardening group, plus get all of your charting done and get out of the community by 3 p.m., you may approach invitations with a hurried attitude. Chances are that Susie Resident isn't going to want to plant flowers with you then either.

Your attitude towards residents affects their decision to participate in an event or program. Make a conscious effort to be encouraging and sincere. Sometimes, especially on a bad or stressful day, it might be difficult to muster up the positive attitude that your residents need to hear in a genuine way. Trust me, your residents will know from a mile away if you do not sincerely want them to attend the activity. Your attitude is important, so be aware of it.

Discussion

Have you ever had a bad day that might have spilled into your workday?

Do you have tricks on how to "fake it" with a positive attitude at work when you're having a busy or bad day?

Activity

Let's try the activity again. Split into pairs. Person #2, tell your partner that it is time to go to gardening group, and be pleasant and excited. All I want you to say is, "It's time for gardening group." Be sure to look in their eyes, smile, and be warm. Person #1, are you going to go to gardening group? Let's share how your reactions are different from the first time.

There's a lot to be said for a warm and friendly attitude, especially when inviting someone to a program. When you're gathering residents for a group or reminding them of an upcoming event, you're setting the tone for the whole interaction. Be sure to call them by name, get down to their physical level if they are not standing, look them in the eyes, sound genuinely excited about the group and about their participation — and smile! Chances are high that they'll come with you and enjoy the program.

Let's go back to Susie as an example. Susie's assessment says that she has been an avid gardener throughout her life. When you invite her to attend, be sure to mention that you know that about her. Try this, "Hi Susie! We are headed out to the garden today for gardening group. I've never really had a green thumb and could sure use your help since you're an experienced gardener. Shall we go?"

Discussion

How do you use the resident assessment and the resident's history to help you know who to invite to programs?

Where do we keep the resident assessment forms so that you can take a look at them?

Now let's take a look at attitudes while leading programs. I have a great Bingo example to show you.

Activity

Process: *Instructor passes out Bingo cards to each person in the inservice and begins to call Bingo numbers. Calling should be done in a friendly way.*

Really quickly, people are going to ask you how they are supposed to mark their numbers. Once they do, the instructor acts annoyed and says, "Well, sorry that I made a mistake. I'll get the markers." Instructor gets the markers, tosses them on the table, and says, "There. Is that better?"

Instructor continues to call a few more numbers and then stops. Ask the group if they had fun at Bingo. They will mention that you were short with them when you went to get the markers.

I want to thank you for your honest responses about my annoyance. That's the point I want to make. A happy group leader can sometimes become derailed during an activity. While this Bingo example was a little dramatic, you can see the point. Acting annoyed or hurried during an event can turn the program sour. We need to be sure to maintain a positive attitude during the program, even if we make a mistake or when a resident is testing our patience.

Discussion

What do you do when a resident comes to a group with complaints?

Can any of you share a time when a resident complained during a program? How did you handle it?

Another way to dampen the mood of a group is to call attention to a resident. Let's go back to Susie, our gardener. She made it to gardening group. However, Susie stays quiet and isn't answering any of the flower trivia questions you've prepared for the beginning of the group. You would like to get her involved, but you respect her decision to stay quiet and observe. Singling her or any other resident out for not responding to questions will not help the mood of the group.

How you present yourself and what your body language says is often more important than the content of the program you are leading. If you are warm, sincere, and not hurried, your residents will enjoy your program even more!

Discussion

Do any of our residents prefer to observe groups instead of actively participate?

Are any of you shy and prefer not to speak in large groups? How do you feel when you're called on during a group to speak? (You can even use how you feel about this question to help you answer.)

What are some ideas of how to get shy residents to participate without making it seem frightening or intimidating?

So that's the presentation on the importance of approach and attitude during invitation and facilitation of groups. Let's think about how we can apply these ideas to our programming.

Discussion

How can we apply this inservice to our department and our groups?

How can we use this information to improve working relationships between the groups who are here today?

Inservice #1
Excitement Is Contagious

Inservice Overview: How to get the attention, and keep the attention, of residents in a group setting. How to motivate residents to attend programs. How to encourage residents to get involved in a group activity.

Presented by: ______________________________

Date: ______________________________

Start Time: ______________________________

End Time: ______________________________

NAME	DEPARTMENT

2.
The Dimensions of Wellness

How the eight dimensions of wellness provide ideas for improving programs.

Topics
Introduction, definition, and brief examples of programming within the dimensions of wellness (physical, occupational, intellectual, social, emotional, spiritual, environmental, and cultural).

Who to Invite
Activity staff, CNA staff, nursing staff, department managers.

Time
About 60 minutes, more if detailed discussions of how to meet needs are included. Detailed programming discussions are probably more appropriate as separate meetings.

Supplies
Inservice sign-in sheet.
Dimension of Me worksheet (at the end of this chapter), one copy for each person.

Co-presenters
CNA supervisor, nursing supervisor.

Content Reminders
Feel free to add your own examples and experience.

"Wellness" is a buzzword that has been around for about a decade. Living a balanced life has been a topic of conversation for those who serve the aging population as well. In fact, the International Council on Active Aging (ICAA) recognizes the seven dimensions of wellness that we are going to discuss today, and even adds another dimension. The fact is this: professionals are realizing that health involves much more than the physical component. From a recreation or activities standpoint, we may see that point a bit more easily than our clinical counterparts. For example, someone who is in a wheelchair or someone who is living with cancer can still have a high quality of life and be "well."

In order to help professionals understand wellness a bit more, researchers and authors created dimensions of wellness. Someone who is living a balanced life should be able to meet each dimension of wellness. Knowing these dimensions can help us develop better programs for our residents. We can also apply the dimensions to our own lives. Let's start by reviewing the seven generally accepted dimensions of wellness, and then we will cover the eighth dimension that is recognized by the ICAA.

These dimensions are listed on the *Dimensions of Me* worksheet. After we talk about each dimension, we'll write a list of what a person might do to achieve wellness in that dimension. As you fill in your ideas for each dimension of wellness, think about what you do in your own life to meet this dimension. You might have many actions under each dimension, or you might notice that some dimensions are lacking in your own life. This is common for everyone, including our residents. This worksheet is strictly for your use, so please be honest as you are filling it out. No one else here will see it. However, if you feel up to sharing during our discussions, that would be great. Now, let's go through the dimensions one by one.

Physical Wellness

The first dimension of wellness might be the easiest for people to relate to and define — the physical dimension. Having physical wellness means that you can get through your activities of daily living without stress. You are free from disease or manage any disease you have successfully. You are strong and fit. Physical wellness activities or best practices might be exercise, eating well, stretching, getting annual physician checkups, getting plenty of rest, and/or taking medications properly. Think about your own life — let's take a few minutes for you to jot down on your worksheet what you do for your own physical wellness and some other things a person might do.

Discussion

What surprised you about your own physical wellness?

If one of our residents has diabetes, could they still be physically well? How?

What are some examples of programs that we offer here that meet the physical dimension of wellness?

Social Wellness

The dimension that we will cover next is something that we are pretty good at in activities — the social dimension. Having a healthy social dimension of wellness means that you are fostering good and supportive relationships in your life. The key word for social wellness is "positive" — positive relationships are needed, not negative relationships. Relationships that make you feel comfortable, encouraged, supported, loved, and even challenged contribute to your social dimension of wellness. Scheduling a regular "girls' or guys' night" to connect with your friends, joining a book club, or having dinner with family are all ways to stay socially well.

While meeting in person is the best-case scenario, keeping in touch via the phone also helps in maintaining social wellness. While some will say that online contact meets social wellness needs, I would like to think that being able to see my best friend and give her a hug is a lot more personal than just shooting her an email. However, that said, the internet does give us multiple ways to connect with friends and family around the world. I think that we just need to be sure that the social media posts are connecting with people in a real way, and not just videos of cats or political rants. What about you? Take a few minutes to write down how things in your life meet your social dimension of wellness and add other things a person might do.

Discussion

When you take a look at your worksheet, are you connecting to people in person or mostly online? Do you experience a difference in the closeness depending on the type of media?

Do you think that connecting via social media maintains social wellness? Does it matter what the content of the posts is? Why?

What are some challenges our residents face in meeting the social dimension? What types of programs do we currently offer to meet these challenges?

What are some examples of programs that we offer here that meet the social dimension of wellness?

Intellectual Wellness

Let's review the intellectual dimension next. This dimension has everything to do with brainpower. Learning new things and keeping the brain active are the hallmark for this dimension, which goes above and beyond crossword puzzles and word searches. Learning a new hobby, traveling somewhere new, and learning a foreign language are all good examples of ways to improve your intellectual dimension of wellness. We have all heard the phrase, "Use it or lose it." This applies directly to intellectual wellness. Turn to your worksheet now and jot down ways that you stay intellectually fit and other ways another person might use.

Discussion

Can a resident with dementia be intellectually "well"? How?

This dimension can be a little weak for many people. How does yours look?

If we teach residents a new dance step during exercise class, does that count as the physical dimension or intellectual dimension or both? Why?

Spiritual Wellness

Next up is the spiritual dimension of wellness. While it is easy to chalk this dimension up to church activities — and those can be a valid part of it — it is not all about singing hymns. The spiritual dimension has a lot to do with connection and peace, finding a meaningful way for each person to connect with the human spirit. Whether attending religious services or studying the holy book, gardening, meditating, praying, or practicing yoga, this dimension can look very different for each of us. What does your spiritual dimension look like? Jot it down and take a few minutes to think about it. Also list ways another person might use to have spiritual wellness.

Discussion

If a resident we serve is Buddhist, are we responsible for helping maintain their spiritual dimension of wellness? How could we start doing that?

Why would gardening be an activity in the spiritual dimension for some people? Can you think of other activities that might be spiritual for some?

Did your spiritual dimension include both religious-based and non-religious-based activities?

Are there any residents right now whose spiritual needs aren't being met? What needs do they have? We'll make a note of these so we can figure out ways to meet them during planning sessions.

Emotional Wellness

The next dimension of wellness that we'll cover is the emotional dimension. Knowing about ourselves and knowing how to cope in a healthy manner with stressful situations are important for us to maintain a healthy emotional state. Joining and attending a support group, seeing a counselor, or participating in regular stress management activities are ways that we can have a healthy emotional dimension of wellness. Like our spiritual dimension activities, each person will have a wide variety of ways to stay emotionally healthy. Your stress outlet might be running, or it might be painting. Whatever it is, as long as it helps you cope and helps you know yourself better, it is meeting your emotional dimension. What are some of your activities? Let's take a few minutes to write down yours and other activities that someone else might find beneficial.

Discussion

What kind of activities or services can we provide to residents to help them maintain a healthy emotional dimension of wellness?

Running was listed as an example of an activity for a healthy emotional dimension for some. Why wouldn't running be considered in the physical dimension? Or would it?

Our jobs can sometimes be emotionally draining. How do you cope?

Some types of coping are not healthy. Think about overindulging in alcohol or smoking. What are some other coping methods that might not be a positive contribution to physical health for us or our residents?

Occupational Wellness

The next dimension to discuss is occupational wellness. Sometimes you will hear this referred to as the "purposeful" dimension, as it involves contributing to a job or a greater purpose. For people who are working, this dimension involves making sure that they like their job and maintain a healthy work/life balance. For people, like our residents, who are no longer working, this dimension might be full of volunteer opportunities or other ways that they can contribute in a meaningful way to a purpose bigger than themselves.

Concrete things for our residents might be participating in Resident Council, helping activities set up for an event, folding napkins for the dining room, intergenerational interactions with school children, or making contributions during our Social Committee meetings. For you, it might be making sure that you take your vacation days, posting an inspirational quote near the time clock, or making a folder for thank-you notes from residents that you can pull out to look at when you are feeling drained. For some of us, our occupational dimension might be met because we just truly love serving seniors and, most times, we love coming to work in the morning. Take a few minutes to write down your thoughts on this.

Discussion

Why would it be important for our residents to have opportunities to meet the occupational dimension?

How would you describe this dimension in your own words?

What are some volunteer opportunities that we have available, or could create, to offer to residents who need help in this dimension?

Environmental Wellness

Our final dimension of the seven is environmental wellness. This dimension focuses on the environment that we live in and our impact on and responsibility to it. Being confident that your environment offers clean water and clean air is one of the first steps to environmental wellness. Once you are in a safe and clean environment, you can focus on your responsibility and actions to keeping it that way. Gardening, recycling, or upcycling, or even visiting a local park or forest preserve can contribute positively to your environmental wellness. Let's take a moment to fill out our worksheets with ideas for ourselves and others.

> **Discussion**
>
> Our residents might have a very small environment right now — their room, our community. How can we give them opportunities to work on their environmental wellness?
>
> How can we keep residents assured of a safe and clean environment here?
>
> What do you do to make your personal environment — your home, your town, your world — better?

Cultural Wellness

I wanted to be sure that we covered the seven most-recognized dimensions of wellness. However, after reading more about the ICAA's eighth dimension, I felt we should cover it, too. The eighth dimension of wellness is cultural wellness. This dimension of wellness honors the past and looks towards the future. It recognizes traditions and cultures that are important to us. Activities such as making our grandma's stuffing recipe on Thanksgiving, attending ethnic celebrations, and simply appreciating the diversity of the world that we live in contribute to our cultural wellness. On your worksheet jot down ways that you and others can keep culturally well.

> **Discussion**
>
> What do you think of the eighth dimension of cultural wellness?
>
> How do you think this dimension applies to our residents?
>
> How can we offer opportunities to our residents that are tailored to this cultural dimension?
>
> What are some ways that you celebrate your culture or the diversity of others?

Overall Wellness

In order to be balanced and well, we should be able to think of activities that we do for each dimension. These dimensions will change from time to time, and we might find that we are weaker in one area in our 30s but weaker in another area when we are in our 80s. Each dimension is important and each dimension helps shape our quality of life.

Sometimes activities can overlap dimensions and that is great. For example, we mentioned in our discussion of the emotional dimension that running might be a stress relief as well as something that keeps us physically healthy. Line dancing would fall into physical wellness, as well as social wellness and intellectual wellness. Let's take a moment to look at wellness as a whole.

> **Discussion**
>
> What is wellness? Is it different from health?
>
> Can you have poor physical health but still be "well" in other ways? Do we have any residents that are like that?
>
> Were you surprised about anything on your worksheet?

As we program for our residents and provide services, let's make an effort to think about each of these dimensions of wellness. It is our responsibility to be sure that our residents have a varied and balanced menu of activity choices here in our community.

Dimensions of Me

Physical Dimension

Social Dimension

Intellectual Dimension

Spiritual Dimension

Emotional Dimension

Occupational Dimension

Environmental Dimension

Cultural Dimension

Inservice #2
The Dimensions of Wellness

Inservice Overview: Introduction, definition, and brief examples of programming within the dimensions of wellness (physical, occupational, intellectual, social, emotional, spiritual, environmental, and cultural)

Presented by: ______________________________

Date: ______________________________

Start Time: ______________________________

End Time: ______________________________

NAME	DEPARTMENT

3.
Our Activity Calendar

Looking at the activity calendar to make sure it covers all eight dimensions of wellness.

Topics
Reviewing the community's activity calendar in relation to the eight dimensions of wellness.

Who to Invite
Activity staff, CNA staff who lead programs with residents, department heads, marketing staff.

Time
30-40 minutes.

Supplies
Inservice sign-in sheet.
Copies of your current activity calendar.
Eight colors of markers or highlighters at each table.
Chart that specifies which color of marker goes with each dimension of wellness.

Review Material
Dimensions of wellness from Inservice 2.

Content Reminders
Use lots of real-life examples and encourage brainstorming to work as a team to make the calendar better.

In an earlier inservice we talked about the dimensions of wellness — physical, social, emotional, spiritual, intellectual, occupational, environmental, and cultural — and how it is vital at any age for everyone to have a balance of each in his or her life in order to be "well." This inservice is an opportunity to learn more about how our activity offerings and calendar meet the requirements of the dimensions of wellness.

Discussion

Let's start by going over each of the dimensions of wellness. Who would like to describe the physical dimension? Social? Emotional? Spiritual? Intellectual? Occupational? Environmental? Cultural?

In order to promote balanced wellness for our residents, the activities department needs to offer a balanced activity calendar. We also must provide independent leisure materials so residents can become involved in the dimensions of wellness in our community.

Today we will focus solely on our activity calendar and the programs that we offer to our residents. It is my hope that we will be honest with one another as we look at the calendar. We can use this training as an opportunity to take a look at what we are doing well and what we need to improve. In order to provide the best programs and services to our residents, we need to do an activity calendar review on a regular basis. In order to make our calendar evaluation well rounded, it is best if we can gather staff from each department to provide input.

Discussion

Before we look at our activity calendar in detail, how well do you think that we meet the dimensions of wellness for our residents?

Even though we plan our calendar three to five weeks ahead of time, please keep in mind that our activity calendar should be somewhat fluid. Our March calendar this year might look very different from our March calendar last year — and it should. Our calendar should be based on resident interests, abilities, and preferences. Our residents last year might have needed different things than the residents this year. Our calendar should reflect that. Further, our calendar should reflect not only our community but also the greater community around us. Our calendar should look different month to month as our community offers different opportunities and as the world changes around us.

Activity

Today we are going to look at the calendar for this month, for our current residents. Each table has eight colors of markers or highlighters. You are going to use a different color to highlight each activity that meets a certain dimension of wellness. For example, on your calendar, use the color pink to highlight each physical activity and yellow for each intellectual activity. There is a chart to let you know which color to use for each dimension of wellness.

You can mark an activity with more than one color if it covers more than one dimension of wellness. Pick a primary dimension for each activity.

Once you are done with all of the dimensions of wellness, tally up on the side of your calendar how many activities we have for each dimension, using the primary dimension you chose for the activity.

Now that everyone is done, let's talk about it. Let's keep in mind that "balanced" does not mean "equal." We do not need 20 physical activities, 20 spiritual activities, 20 environmental activities, etc. Instead we need a nice balance of all of the dimensions of wellness throughout our calendar.

Discussion

First, take a look at your calendar. Do you think it looks balanced?

What are dimension are we great at?

What dimension are we not so great at? How can we work together to fix that?

What are five activity ideas for two dimensions that we are most lacking in?

Are there any activities that we are currently offering that we shouldn't be doing based on resident interest or preferences?

Activities can definitely have more than one dimension, based on the resident and what they get out of it. For example, if Mrs. Jones loves craft group because she gets to sit next to her girlfriends and visit, then crafts are social for her. However, if Mrs. Anderson loves craft group because it relaxes her to create things, then craft group is emotional for her. Gardening might be physical for some and spiritual for others. Each of our residents gets something different out of each group we run. I think that is exciting — it's awesome that we can make a difference in the wellbeing of our residents in different ways, just by offering programming!

Discussion

Some of you might have found it hard to pick only one dimension for a certain activity. Did any of you find that?

Can you give us examples of activities that you couldn't decide on?

I hope this exercise has empowered you to look at our calendar and our activities in a different way. You should feel that you are able to explain this to residents, staff, and/or family members. It will help them understand the value of activities and how participation can positively affect our residents in a variety of ways.

Inservice #3
Our Activity Calendar

Inservice Overview: Reviewing the community's activity calendar in relation to the eight dimensions of wellness.

Presented by: ______________________________

Date: ______________________________

Start Time: ______________________________

End Time: ______________________________

NAME	DEPARTMENT

4.
Leisure Assessments and Inventories

Why assessments and inventories are important aspects of program planning and leading groups.

Topics
Review of assessment tools that the community uses. Description of how assessment tools can be helpful when leading groups.

Who to Invite
Activity staff, CNA staff who lead activity programs, care plan coordinator.

Time
20-30 minutes, plus about 10 minutes for each blank and completed assessment you cover.

Supplies
Inservice sign-in sheet.
Blank copies of your community's assessment and leisure inventory tools.
Copies of a completed assessment and inventory. These must be destroyed after the inservice to protect the privacy of the resident.

Co-presenters
Care plan coordinator.

Review Material
Community-specific tools and information about assessments.
Federal, state, and facility regulations regarding assessment and documentation for residents.

Content Reminders
Use lots of resident-specific examples to make this training even more meaningful.

Completing our activity assessment and inventory is a critical step in getting to know our residents and figuring out how to best program for them. Our assessment process is kind of like putting pieces of a puzzle together. We are trying to find out what our residents love doing, what makes them feel purposeful and happy, and what is currently blocking them from doing the things that they love. The assessment and inventory can seem like a lot of paperwork for us to complete in a timely fashion, and it is — but it is also a wonderful way to learn about our residents!

Regulations say that we need to assess all residents new to our community.

Tell participants what your state says specifically for your particular license type.

We also have to reassess them at different times during their stay, and when they have a significant change.

Review these times with your participants in regards to your state and license.

We are essentially taking a snapshot of our resident, finding out where they are now. What can they still do? What do they like to do? With our assessment process, we are also finding out about what they were like. Sometimes, we have to remind ourselves that we are meeting our residents in the later years of their life. They may have had 90 or more years of experiences, memories, laughter, and hobbies. What did they do for a job before they retired? What is their family situation like?

Once we get all of this background and current information, we can sit down and figure out how to best serve this new resident. If our new resident was once a second-grade teacher and said that having kids around makes her happy, let's figure out a way to get her involved with a Girl Scout troop's intergenerational activity. If a resident has had a stroke and cannot use her left hand, let's remember that and sit near her to help her complete a craft project she loves doing. If another resident says that he has always preferred being a "homebody" and has never been one for making new friends and attending new activities, let's find a way to meet him in his room and not pressure him to get involved in an activity with lots of people that might make him uncomfortable.

While we cannot get to know all about our new or returning residents through our assessment process, we can make a good start. Remember, if the resident is confused, we still need to attempt the assessment. Perhaps trying the next day or trying in the morning as opposed to the evening might help the resident's clarity. The same applies to a new or returning resident who is sleeping. Let's make every effort to reach that resident and keep trying to find a time when they are awake. We can always consult with the family contact to get the answers to our questions, but the resident is our best source of information.

Discussion

How do you use our resident assessments and inventories right now?

Are they getting you the kind of information you need to program for residents?

Let's go ahead and take a look at our blank assessment and inventory form.

Discussion

Process: *Pass out blank forms to participants and point out different sections as well as how each section of the forms can assist with program planning or invitations. Add your own experience with filling out the form and roadblocks that you might have encountered to filling it out. Answer any questions that they might have about the forms.*

Where do we keep the completed assessment forms? Are you able to access the forms so that you can review them on each resident?

What system do we have in place to assure that you read over assessments on new and returning residents?

Now let's take a look at an assessment that is completed. This is one of our newer residents and I thought it would be good for you to see one completed.

Discussion

Process: *Pass out a completed assessment and inventory to each participant. Allow a few minutes for participants to read the information and then lead a discussion on the content.*

Is there anything in the assessment that surprises you?

How will the resident's medical diagnosis affect programming or invitations to events?

Let's brainstorm on activities that the resident might enjoy, thinking about group programs as well as independent pursuits in the resident's room.

Why do you think it is important for us to reassess our residents on a regular basis and when there is a significant change?

If we see that a resident once enjoyed crocheting but now can no longer do it because of medical reasons, how should we respond? What should we offer?

How do we get to know our residents, besides the assessment and inventory process?

When you get to know a resident, does it change the way you invite them to programs? How?

Trainer note: If you are looking for another way to get your staff involved with reading the assessments for residents, find a few interesting facts about residents that are listed in their assessments. Give each person two facts without the resident names as they leave the training — different facts for each attendee. Tell them that if they find out which residents are described and come up with two more interesting facts about residents, they will get a prize. Examples include: Which of our residents used to be a lawyer? Which of our residents lived in Spain for a few years? Be sure that the information is something that is found in the residents' assessments.

Inservice #4

Why Leisure Assessments and Inventories Are So Important

Inservice Overview: Review of assessment tools that community uses. Description of how they can be helpful when leading groups

Presented by:______________________________

Date:______________________________

Start Time:______________________________

End Time:______________________________

NAME	DEPARTMENT

5.
Using the Participation Record

Using the participation record for more than just attendance during group interactions.

Topics
Review of how and when to use the participation record, how to look for trends, and how that can affect our choice of programming.

Who to Invite
Activity staff, CNA staff who lead activity programs.

Time
20-30 minutes, plus about 10 minutes to discuss each resident participation record.

Supplies
Inservice sign-in sheet.
Blank copies of your community's participation record.
Copies of two or three completed records of current residents.

Co-presenters
Staff with experience using participation records.

Review Material
Community-specific tools.
State-specific regulatory information.

Content Reminders
Use lots of resident-specific examples and discussion to make this training even more meaningful.

Our participation records are an important part of charting on each resident. Before we get into why charting participation is so important for us here at our community, let's review our state regulations that pertain to the record.

Review your state-specific regulations regarding the participation record.

So we know that the participation record is an important part of how we meet regulations. But we can use the information that we collect for much more. Before we get into how we can use the records for watching for trends and behaviors, let's review how to complete our forms.

Activity

Process: *Walk through your form with your team and talk about the correct way to complete the information. If you use electronic charting, be sure to walk participants through that process as well. Have more veteran members of your staff to help out with this part. While it might seem redundant going over this information, it is worth revisiting for this inservice. Feel free to use resident-specific examples and information to make the review more relevant.*

We can use our participation records to track resident interests and preferences. Let's take a look at an example in regards to sleeping during programs. For example, if we are able to see from the record that one of our residents always falls asleep during morning exercise, we need to investigate further.

Discussion

Should we be working with nursing to have this resident take a nap after breakfast?

Can we engage even more with this resident so that he doesn't fall asleep?

Could we ask the resident to help us lead the exercise group or sit him closer to us to encourage him to stay awake?

Does the resident like exercise — perhaps he is falling asleep because he is bored?

We can also look at information regarding behaviors. If we notice that a resident consistently leaves programming early, we could investigate further and see that she only leaves late-afternoon activities. We could then ask ourselves a few questions.

Discussion

Is she leaving the program early because she is anxious or restless?

Is this a new behavior?

Should we discuss this with nursing staff? Is she leaving because she is bored?

Can we offer her a more engaged role during the program to keep her participating?

If we notice trends on the participation record and follow up by trying new things with the resident, we can hopefully engage residents better based on their personal preferences and interests. If you notice a trend, let's be sure to talk about it as a group. One trend worth noting is an activity or intervention that is working quite well with a resident. Another trend is an activity or intervention that is a complete failure. We need to know it all so that we can best serve our residents. Trying new interventions might end up in changing the activity plan of care for the resident.

Now, let's take a look at participation records from a few of our residents.

Discussion

Are there any trends that you can see here?

Based on the trends, what are the problem areas we find?

How can we improve the overall care plan and specific interventions for this resident?

To summarize, we can see that participation records are a valuable part of our work. The question to ask now is how we can use them most effectively.

Discussion

How can our team make an effort to review our participation records on a regular basis to look for trends?

Is there any way to make our charting in the record more effective or efficient?

Inservice #5
Using the Participation Record

Inservice Overview: Review of how and when to use the participation record, how to look for trends, and how that can affect our choice of programming

Presented by:______________________________

Date:______________________________

Start Time:______________________________

End Time:______________________________

NAME	DEPARTMENT

6.
Activities-Regulations Jeopardy

Jeopardy-based challenge to improve understanding of state and federal regulations.

Topics
Review of state and federal activities regulations, done in a Jeopardy format.

Who to Invite
Activity staff, CNA staff who lead programs with residents.

Time
30-40 minutes.

Supplies
Inservice sign-in sheet.
Prepared questions hung on the wall under Jeopardy-like categories (suggestions below).
Hershey's Kisses or other treats to pass out for correct answers.
A "fabulous prize" for the winning team, such as lunch certificates, fun pens/pencils, etc.

Review Material
Regulations from your state and federal guidelines.
Community-specific information.

Content Reminders
This training is best done just before your annual state survey window. It is a way for you to communicate and reinforce regulations that your staff need to be aware of, in a fun and interactive way.

How to play:

- Divide the group of participants into two or three teams.
- Have five or six categories taped to the wall, with five questions under each.
- Each question is worth points (100, 200, 300, 400, 500).
- Flip a coin to see which team goes first.
- A team picks a question and answers it. If they are correct, they pick another question; if they are incorrect, it is the next team's turn.
- Each member of the team gets a Hershey kiss for the correct answers.
- Teams are responsible for keeping track of their points.

- The team with the most points at the end of the game wins a fabulous prize.

Extras

- You can choose to do a "double jeopardy" round with more questions, if you have time.
- You do not have to phrase information in the form of a statement if you do not want to.
- You might want to consider allowing another team to "steal" the points if a team answers incorrectly.

How to develop your questions:

- Choose your categories. Ideas might include Safety, Food, Calendar, Leading Groups, One-on-Ones, Confidentiality and Privacy, and Environment.
- Choose your questions. Here are a few ideas to get you started. Check with your federal, state and community guidelines for accuracy when you are completing yours.
    - Safety: What does PASS stand for in regards to fire extinguishers? (Pull the pin, Aim, Squeeze, and Sweep)
    - Food: Who can feed a resident with feeding precautions during an activity? (A CNA or nurse)
    - Calendar: Who is our Resident Council President?
    - Leading Groups: If an activity is scheduled to begin at 9 a.m., what time should it really start? (9 a.m.)
    - One-on-ones: Where do we keep our one-on-one list and interventions?
    - Confidentiality and Privacy: What should you do before entering a resident's room? (Knock on the door and wait for permission to enter.)
    - Environment: If your environment for your group is very loud due to chatty CNAs at the nursing station, what should you do? (Ask them to quiet down.)
- Assign points to each question.
- Write questions on index cards or half sheets of paper. You can also type them.
- After you play the game, keep the questions and category topics together in a file for you to pull out and use next time.

Inservice #6
Activities Regulations Jeopardy

Inservice Overview: Review of state and federal activities regulations for a SNF community, done in a Jeopardy format.

Presented by:______________________________

Date:______________________________

Start Time:______________________________

End Time:______________________________

NAME	DEPARTMENT

7.
Basics of One-on-One Activities

Making sure that one-on-one visits meet the needs of the residents.

Topics
Review of one-on-one visits, requirements, reasons, and charting.

Who to Invite
Activity staff, CNA staff who lead programs with residents, care plan coordinator, volunteers who regularly perform one-on-one visits.

Time
30 minutes, plus time to discuss plans for residents on the revised one-on-one visit list.

Supplies
Inservice sign-in sheet.

Review Material
State and federal guidelines for one-on-ones.
Community-specific policies for one-on-ones.
If you are unsure of the guidelines, contact your consultant or mentor in the area.

Content Reminders
Use lots of resident-specific examples and discussion to make this training even more meaningful.

Sometimes, one-on-ones can be confusing. Who gets them? Who doesn't get them? What happens during the visit? How long does the visit take? All of these questions can cause confusion and frustration. Let's work together during this training to really dig into the regulations and find out how we can serve our residents better through appropriate and efficient one-on-ones.

The idea of the one-on-one visit is a really good, resident-centered idea. If a resident does not join groups and does not get visitors, we should be concerned. There is a chance that the resident is isolated and not thriving from a social perspective. A successful one-on-one visit is done by people who are trained in that resident's interests and preferences. They reach out and connect with the resident throughout the week. That all sounds great, right?

However, somehow along the way, the one-on-one visit has gotten a bit of a bad rap. Lists of residents who need one-on-ones can be much too long. Visits may not accomplish what is intended.

The easiest way to get started is to first decide who needs the one-on-one visits. Here are the guidelines for our community.

Talk about your specific policies and regulations regarding who gets one-on-ones.

You will notice that a resident needs a one-on-one when the following is true:

- Is not involved in consistent group programming.
- Does not get any visitors.
- Does not participate in any independent leisure.
- Cannot pursue leisure without some assistance.

We need think about how many residents currently meets that description.

Discussion

What kind of resident currently gets on the one-on-one list?

An effective one-on-one program starts with charting. When we sit down and take a look at the care plan, the interest survey and assessment, and the participation records for our residents, it can sometimes seem that the resident is not doing anything at all. However, that is often not true. Many things a resident does can be left out of the charts. We must remember to chart all that our residents do for a truer picture of their leisure pursuits.

Discussion

How does our community record resident participation in the charts?

Do we chart non-group activities?

Let's look at some examples:

If a resident gets visitors consistently, where is that charted and who can chart it?

If a resident loves watching her daytime soap operas, where is that charted and who can chart it?

If a resident naps all morning long (by preference), but stays up chatting online late at night, where is that charted and who can chart it?

Are there other similar situations that are specific to our community and how do we chart them?

Once we have an accurate view of the resident's leisure pursuits and preferences, during all times of the day, we are able to determine the need for a one-on-one visit. Residents who can make their own decisions about activities typically do not need a structured one-on-one visit. Let's consider Mr. Smith. He is alert and oriented. He refuses activity invitations. And he tells you in no uncertain terms that he just wants to stay in his room and read the newspaper. Mr. Smith probably does not need a one-on-one visit. Now, that does not mean that we should never stop by to say hello. It's all right to check in with a social visit with Mr. Smith. All we're saying is that he can decide when and if he would like to participate in groups.

On the flip side, let's think about Mr. Jones. He is unable to leave his bed without nursing assistance. He is usually put in bed unless at meals. He is unable to pursue any leisure of his own. And he has no one who visits him regularly. We should be interacting on a one-on-one basis with him.

Part of our job is to develop a list of residents who need structured one-on-one visits. This list should be relatively short.

Discussion

Which of our residents need one-on-one visits?

Having the list, we need to develop an actual schedule of visits.

Review policy and regulations regarding timing of visits. Most regulations state that visits must be on a set schedule. The time for these visits should also be on the activity calendar.

Probably the most important aspect of the one-on-one visit is the content of the visit itself. These visits are not social visits. You are not just stopping in to say hi and chat about the weather. Instead, these visits are based on resident preferences and abilities, and are listed on the care plan. Each resident will have a different plan and different interventions during the visits. The resident's one-on-one visit plan will have ideas that were written specifically for that resident, based on the resident's abilities and interests. Don't veer from this list of activities when you choose what to do with your time together.

You should enter each visit prepared with supplies specific to that resident. Never walk into a one-on-one visit unprepared. Instead, make the most of your time with the resident by bringing in a variety of props and materials to make your interaction as valuable as possible. An intervention or activity may not work for the resident any longer. Be sure to bring it to my attention so that we can talk about it and alter the care plan as needed.

Use this time to review policy and regulations regarding content of visits. Give concrete examples of what a one-on-one visit should look like for specific residents.

Discussion

Where do we keep our one-on-one list?

Where do we keep our one-on-one supplies?

How do we chart one-on-one visits?

Since one-on-one visits are not just social visits, you will need to consult with one another, with me, and with the resident and family to find out what types of activities you could do together. Trial and error will be necessary as you find out what works. Is depends on the resident. A few ideas might be reading a book aloud or together, doing a Bible study together, playing a game, listening to recordings of old baseball games, or knitting together. If the resident is lower functioning, your one-on-one visit might include listening to hymns, giving a hand massage for relaxation, or looking at photo albums. Let's look at specific residents who need one-on-one programs.

Discussion

For each resident who was added to the list: Brainstorm together for more interventions or new things to try. Be sure that everyone knows where the supplies are for each one-on-one visit.

For residents who currently have one-on-one programs: Pull care plans and review the interventions listed to determine if they are still appropriate.

Inservice #7
Basics of One-on-One Activities

Inservice Overview: Review of one-on-one visits, requirements, reasoning, and charting
Presented by: ____________________
Date:____________________
Start Time:____________________
End Time:____________________

NAME	DEPARTMENT

8.
Independent Leisure

Using independent leisure activities with residents.

Topics
How to meet the needs of residents who sometimes prefer to pursue leisure independently outside of a group setting.

Who to Invite
Activity staff, CNA staff who lead programs with residents, care plan coordinator, nursing shift leaders.

Time
30-40 minutes.

Supplies
Inservice sign-in sheet.

Review Material
State-specific information regarding regulations about independent leisure pursuits.

Content Reminders
It is important that the participants leave with a full understanding of where independent leisure pursuit materials are located and how to access them, no matter the time of day.
Use lots of resident-specific examples and discussion to make this training even more meaningful.

Not everyone is a big group person. Not everyone is a small group person. We have residents who are extroverts and love being a part of a group. They like interacting with people. We also have residents who are introverts and prefer more time in their day away from the bustling noises and business of the dining room and therapy room. Our goal is an activity program with opportunities for both group interactions and for independent leisure pursuits. All residents should have the mix they desire.

What exactly is independent leisure? It is activities that you complete on your own, during your down time or another time of your choosing. Independent leisure requires no one else but you. It typically has benefits of stress relief and independence. Think about your own life. While you are probably "go, go, go" at work and then at home again, you still have pockets of time in your day when you are doing activities or hobbies alone. If you are introverted, you will find that you feel drained after being around groups of people. Then your independent leisure might help you recharge and feel relaxed. If you are extroverted, you tend to recharge from interacting with people, so you might have a little less independent leisure in your life. It might require more of a planned effort. But no matter your personality, independent leisure is important in your life. It is also important in our residents' lives.

Our residents, whether introverted or extroverted, are spending a lot of time around people. Without even leaving the room, our residents interact with nursing staff throughout the day and night. While our team does a great job of respecting privacy, our residents really do live in a communal and medical setting. People are everywhere, all the time. Our residents eat in a dining room with people. They go to therapy sessions with people. They see people in the hallway on the way to their room. And they have group activities with people. Families are visiting. Friends are popping in to say hello. Our residents have almost no down time for independent leisure. Even if they crave it, they have trouble getting it. It might be the most important thing that we can offer them.

Independent leisure can be a relaxing outlet for our residents. It can increase feelings of confidence and empowerment, as the resident sees that he or she can accomplish something without help. In our environment, our residents need help with different aspects of their care and life. It is nice when we are able to find an activity that they can do on their own. Independent leisure also gives our residents the ability to make their own choice. Residents can decide when they would like to pull out their magazine or Bible study. Residents can decide when they would like to start and stop their leisure pursuits. Some residents are actively involved with therapy or other activities throughout the day and evening. They will like choosing when to participate in independent leisure pursuits in their own room, when they are feeling up to it.

Discussion

What do we do with our residents who do not attend group programs?

How do we make sure those residents are still doing activities that they enjoy?

Keep in mind that our residents doing independent activities still might need our help and assistance. We can help find independent leisure materials, make those materials accessible, set up the materials, or put them away. We might also need to educate the residents on why getting involved with independent leisure is important for them and their recovery.

Independent leisure is important for many residents. However, it is not an appropriate intervention for all of them. In order for independent leisure to be successful, the resident needs to be alert and able to tell us what he or she needs and wants. The resident needs to enjoy completing the independent activity. The resident should be able to make the decision of when he or she wants to start and end the activity as well. Some of our residents with dementia might enjoy rolling balls of yarn or polishing silverware as an intervention. While this is independent leisure, the activity staff decide when the resident does the activity.

Discussion

Can you give us an example of a resident who is successful with independent leisure?

What about a resident who would be unsuccessful with independent leisure?

Independent leisure for a resident should be documented in our participation record as well as in the care plan. If you know that a resident plays solitaire in his room every night before dinner, be sure that is in the record and in his care plan. A resident who doesn't attend groups and doesn't have any visitors during the day might seem at risk for isolation. She might seem to require one-on-one visits. This may not be true if she is an avid reader who reads books on her Kindle every day. Her chart needs to note that. Let's be sure that we document independent leisure appropriately and accurately.

Discussion

How do you document independent leisure?

Independent leisure will be what is right for each person. Interests and preferences vary. However, a few examples might be reading, doing crossword puzzles, clipping coupons, emailing, surfing the Internet, playing solitaire, talking on the phone, journaling, painting, drawing, or praying. Even watching TV is all right if it is not done out of boredom or isolation.

Here at our community, it is ultimately our responsibility to be sure that we are doing our best to help residents with their independent leisure. We should have materials available such as the newspaper, current magazines, yarn and knitting or crocheting supplies, crossword puzzle books that we can copy and distribute, books or library access, and art supplies. If we do not have the materials for leisure pursuit, you should be sure to let your supervisor know so that we can get the materials. Also, once you know that a resident enjoys a certain leisure pursuit, be sure that the activity staff and the 24-hour nursing staff know where those materials are. They should be able to access them at any time. For example, a resident may be having a hard night and cannot sleep. The night staff know that the resident loves reading gossip magazines. The activity department keeps a stash in the television cabinet near the resident's room. Then, the nursing staff can grab a few issues and hand them to the resident to enjoy, even if it is at 3 a.m.

Discussion

What are some examples of independent leisure pursuit that we have available here?

What are some materials that we could get to improve our service to our residents?

Where are the materials kept?

How can we be sure they are kept in stock and up-to-date?

Discuss regulations about independent leisure. Discuss community-specific ways to find out about resident preferences and off-hours pursuits. These preferences and off-hours pursuits need to be in the chart and care plan.

Inservice #8
Independent Leisure

Inservice Overview: How to meet the needs of residents who sometimes prefer to pursue leisure independently and not within a group setting.

Presented by:____________________

Date:____________________

Start Time:____________________

End Time:____________________

NAME	DEPARTMENT

9.
Let's Take a Trip

How to lead a successful trip by keeping everyone safe and engaged.

Topics
Policies and procedures regarding outings with residents and best practices for optimum engagement and participation.

Who to Invite
Activity staff, CNA staff who attend outings, resident and family council members interested in helping plan events.

Time
30-40 minutes, longer if time is spent discussing extensive problems with past outings or planning future outings.

Supplies
Inservice sign-in sheet.
Event calendars for the community outside of the facility.

Review Material
State and federal regulations about offering outings.
Community-specific policies and procedures regarding outings.

Content Reminders
Use lots of resident-specific examples and discussion to make this training even more meaningful.

In this inservice we will be looking at offering outings for our residents. To start this discussion, I'd like to hear some of your ideas about the reasons for outings.

Discussion

Why do we do outings with our residents?

Offering outing opportunities to our residents is important for many reasons. Besides the fact that it is required in our regulations, it is a wonderful chance for our residents to get out into the community at large. They can exercise their independence and any new ADL skills they have been working on.

Describe state and federal regulations and community-specific policies related to the reasons for offering outings.

Consider the point of view of our residents. While you and I come to work and then leave work daily to go home, our residents are here in our community all the time. While we have a lovely community, I'm sure that you can appreciate that residents sometimes go a bit stir crazy. Our residents, no matter if they are short term or long term, should be offered the chance to get out into the greater community. They need to check out what is going on in the world beyond our walls. If there is a new restaurant opening, a local festival happening, or a high school musical performance, let's work to connect our residents with it. Our residents do not drive and many do not get out of our community with family members. This isolation from the community around them can lead to depression and decreased feelings of connection. Outings can be a very purposeful and even emotional outlet that our residents need.

For short-term residents, or long-term residents who are working with therapy, our outings can be a wonderful way for them to try out new skills. A resident who is working on lower body strength with therapy might want to practice transferring from a wheelchair to a restaurant chair when we are out. A resident working on fine motor skills after a stroke might want to work on handling money while buying something at a shop. Outings can be a crucial part of physical rehabilitation. Even if there are no other reasons, an outing is a great for getting residents out of their rooms.

Discussion

Currently, how do we choose which residents attend an outing?

Let's review our policies and procedures for outings now. These are the ways we make outings enjoyable and keep residents safe.

Discuss community policies and procedures for trips. Include real life situations that you have encountered as well as a frank and honest conversation about how to keep trips safe. Use about 15-20 minutes just on this topic section to assure that everyone on the team is on the same page and has the same information. Encourage questions and problem solving. Go through the next set of discussion questions.

Discussion

Do we chart who has physician or therapist orders against attending trips? How can we assure that residents who want to attend are able to?

What role do nursing and CNA staff play in helping to assure that residents who are interested in attending trips are able to?

What can CNA and activity staff do prior to the trip to ensure that the trip goes well?

How do we keep our residents safe on trips?

What are some items that we should always bring with us when we attend trips with residents?

In regards to inviting residents, I want us to invite residents to trips that they would enjoy. Some of our residents just love to get out, no matter where we are going, and that is great. Let's just be sure that we are not always inviting the same residents on each of the outings. If there is a trip that you think that a resident might really enjoy, but you are not sure if he or she could handle the trip physically, bring it to me. We can brainstorm together with the nursing staff and the family to see if there is a way for that resident to attend. We should also ask the residents and their families for ideas about events the residents would like to attend. We should never get locked into the idea that we know what is most interesting for our residents, especially when they are right here and we can ask them.

Discussion

Currently, how do we choose which residents attend an outing?

Do we work on trying to get new residents to attend trips, or do we tend to always ask the same ones each time?

How can residents and families help us find and plan events the residents would like to attend?

Once our residents are invited and loaded on the bus, let's remember that the trip to the destination (and back home again) is a crucial time for programming. After all, we do have a captive audience. Best practices include listening to music or audio books that fit the theme of our trip, doing trivia or playing "road trip games," and encouraging conversation between residents and staff. We can talk about the destination, what we think we will see, what we are looking forward to, etc. On the way home, we can talk about what we liked best, what we thought of the experience, etc.

Discussion

How do you keep residents engaged during the trips to and from our destination?

Would anyone here from the nursing or CNA staff like to volunteer to go on trips with us?

What kind of outings should we work on planning over the next six months?

Inservice #9
Let's Take a Trip

Inservice Overview: Policies and procedures regarding outings with residents and best practices for optimum engagement and participation

Presented by:____________________

Date:____________________

Start Time:____________________

End Time:____________________

NAME	DEPARTMENT

10.
How to Work with Volunteers

Successfully working with volunteers within the community's volunteer program.

Topics
Tips on how to successfully work with volunteers and an overview of the community's volunteer program.

Who to Invite
Activity staff, CNA staff who lead programs with residents, volunteer coordinator.

Time
40-50 minutes.

Supplies
Inservice sign-in sheet.

Co-presenters
Volunteer coordinator.

Review Material
Information and guidelines specific to volunteers in your community.
State regulations regarding volunteers.

Content Reminders
Use lots of resident-specific examples and discussion to make this training even more meaningful.

Volunteers are an important part of our community, especially for our activities department. Some volunteers offer long-term, consistent friendship to our residents. Others are like the Girl Scout troop that comes in for a single visit. All of them help to care for our residents. When we work successfully with them, they can alleviate some of our stress.

I realize that sometimes it feels like having a volunteer with you makes your day harder or busier. That's what this inservice is about — working together with volunteers to make your job easier and to better serve our residents.

Discussion

How many volunteers do you think our community currently has?

How do you currently work with volunteers?

Do you think that working with volunteers makes your job harder or easier?

Our volunteers come to us in a variety of ways. Some are church related or community service group related. Some are students and some are people just are looking for a way to give their time to seniors. It is important that you know how these volunteers come to us, how they are chosen to volunteer here, how they are trained, and how they are recognized as being an ancillary part of our team.

Use the next 15-20 minutes to review community-specific information about how your community handles volunteers. Talk about who the volunteer talks to first when they are interested. Talk about the interview, the background checks, and the training that happens prior to the volunteer working with residents. Discuss the difference, if any, in the orientation process for an individual volunteer versus a volunteer group, such as a Boy Scout troop that comes in to sing Christmas carols. Talk about how volunteers sign in and out of your community, how you recognize them at Volunteer Appreciation events, and how you actively recruit and seek volunteers from the greater community.

Ideally, working with a volunteer should lighten your workload a bit and brighten the day of even more residents. Let's review a few best practices on how to work most efficiently and effectively with volunteers, both group and individual.

If you are working with a volunteer group, recognize the goal of the group. Is the group in a long-term relationship with us, or is it a just-one-time group? Is the group made up of adults or children? Knowing the demographics and the intention of the group before you go to meet them can help you mentally prepare for the event.

If your group is coming in for a short-term commitment, there is no need to spend a lot of time showing them where to sign in and out, how to work with certain residents, or what to do in case of an emergency. In this case, it is best to do everything you can to be sure that the residents have a great time in the event and that the volunteers get to interact with the residents and have a good time.

If your volunteer group will be a long-term staple at your community, it is wise to introduce aspects of resident personalities and preferences as well as logistics of the community. Don't feel that you need to tell them everything before they start. You can give them a little more information each time they come by. We don't want to overwhelm our volunteers. Instead, we want them to leave our community feeling energized, appreciated, and excited to come back the next time.

When working with an individual volunteer, spend some of your time getting to know the preferences and expectations of the volunteer. If you know that your volunteer loves knitting, you might want to pair her with a resident who loves knitting, but never leaves her room. What a wonderful one-on-one visitor this volunteer could be for her! If your volunteer is a veteran and likes to talk about that experience, consider having the volunteer lead a small group of veteran residents. Put down a plate of donuts, introduce the volunteer each week, and voila! It is a purposeful and beneficial long-term group for everyone involved. Take your time introducing your volunteers to the residents and community, so that you do not overwhelm them. Also, be very conscious about how you are portraying yourself and the department during your time with them. If you are running around before an event and you seem very frazzled and stressed, you might end up stressing out the volunteer!

Discussion

What is your favorite thing about working with volunteers?

What is something about working with volunteers that frustrates you?

Whether you are working with individuals or groups, it is important that you feel comfortable delegating tasks to them. Our volunteers are here because they want to help, so let them! Give your directions clearly and warmly. For example, you might say, "Jimmy, please go sit by Mr. Anderson, the resident in the red hat. Alice, please go grab those balloons and pass one out to everyone. Susan, you stick with me because I need help passing out the cupcakes." Make sure everyone is involved and has a meaningful part to play.

Discussion

Do you have any tips for delegating tasks to volunteers?

Let's brainstorm. What are some ways (visiting with residents, offering residents snacks or beverages, walking with residents, etc.) that volunteers can be helpful in our department?

Remember, with groups or individuals, you might have to start conversations or interactions with residents for them. It might seem awkward for the volunteers to jump right in and visit with residents, Sometimes volunteers are shy or they might feel put on the spot. Instead, try to have an activity ready, such as checkers, a craft, or something else the resident enjoys. That gives the volunteer and resident something to focus on and work on together. The conversation and relationship will follow.

Finally, before your group or individual volunteer leaves for the day, thank them. Tell them that you appreciate them taking time to come in and help you out today. If possible, try to give them one specific thing that they did that really made a difference or helped you out. For example, "Anna, I haven't seen our resident Joe laugh that hard in a long time. Thank you for spending time with him today!" If you know that you will see the volunteer again soon, give a reminder for their next visit ("I'll see you Friday afternoon!") and send them away with an encouraged heart.

Discussion

How do you thank the volunteers that you work with?

Are there any tasks or activities that volunteers could help out with?

Inservice #10
How to Work with Volunteers

Inservice Overview: Tips on how to successfully work with volunteers and an overview of the community's volunteer program

Presented by:______________________________

Date:______________________________

Start Time:______________________________

End Time:______________________________

NAME	DEPARTMENT

11.
Leading a Successful Reminiscence Group

Successful reminiscence group and why reminiscing is important to our residents.

Topics
Tips on how to lead a successful reminiscence group and why reminiscing is important to our residents.

Who to Invite
Activity staff, CNA staff who lead programs with residents.

Time
30-40 minutes, plus the time spent leading reminiscing groups and creating reminiscing kits.

Supplies
Inservice sign-in sheet.
Examples of reminiscing resources that you have available (*Reminiscence* magazine, photo albums, reminiscing kits, etc.).

Review Material
Examples of different reminiscing tools that you have available at your community. If you find that you are a little bit short on good tools, run out and buy some or put some kits together with things you find on hand.

Content Reminders
This training will be more effective if you are able to demonstrate reminiscing techniques and tools with the group. Watching you model how to lead an effective reminiscing group will be beneficial to your staff. Use this training as an opportunity to introduce the new tools to the staff.

Reminiscence, sometimes called reminiscence therapy, is using objects to trigger memories and discussion from the group or individual that you are working with. Using reminiscence is appropriate for any of our residents, not just those who are living with Alzheimer's disease or other dementias. Many people of all ages have an innate desire to tell their story, to share their memories with others who might be interested. Reminiscence is a way to help residents feel important, empowered, and able to share those memories with you and with one another.

Discussion
What else is part of reminiscence?

The nice thing about reminiscence is that it can be done almost anywhere. You can lead a reminiscing experience for a small group of residents, or you can use it during an individual one-on-one interaction. Once you get the hang of how to facilitate reminiscence, and the tools that make it easier and more personal for the residents, you might find that you are leading reminiscing sessions many times throughout your day. Here are a few things to keep in mind while you are learning how to perfect this art.

Reminiscing is different from regular conversation. When you reminisce, you are headed into the interaction with a goal in mind. In general, your goal will be to evoke memories and communication. However, your goal will be different for each resident, based on the resident's specific situation. Reminiscing is not just open-ended questions, such as tell me about your wedding. It is more about using tools to awaken memories, stories, and details that even the resident might have forgotten.

Reminiscing requires investigation and planning. Before you start your group or individual reminiscing, you need to know your audience. Review the interest survey and assessment about the resident(s) that you will be working with. You want to be prepared with questions and props that will connect with your audience. For example, if your resident grew up in the city of Chicago, you would not bring in a farm-based reminiscence kit. If a resident was never married, a wedding kit would not be an appropriate or effective tool to bring with you. After you get to know your audience and their interests, have some questions and tools with you when you start your interaction.

Another great thing about reminiscing is that it is fluid and flexible. You never know what you will end up talking about at the end of the session. A baseball-themed reminiscing group with your men's club might end up as a session talking about memories of how they proposed to their wives. That is okay. Reminiscing is meant to take you down different roads, all based on the resident memories. The key is to be sure that the residents are leading the conversation.

Reminiscing is not about you. While you might have to share a bit during your interaction to get the conversation flowing, ultimately the group is for the resident's memories. Sometimes, when you have a great story that you want to relate to the group, this can be hard to keep in mind. However, when you are leading a reminiscence group, you are more a facilitator than a leader. It is your role to keep the residents on task and interacting. It is not your role to share more than you need to.

Discussion

When do you use reminiscence?

Do we have reminiscing groups listed on our current calendar?

Tools for reminiscing will look different in each community. The basics include a few photo resources or magazines and themed reminiscing kits that change throughout the year.

Photos are great ways to get conversations going. You can choose to use the photos of the residents themselves. You can also use photos that portray major world events that happened during the younger years of the resident's lives or ones that portray objects that would have been a part of their everyday life.

Reminiscing kits are made of objects that are all related to a certain theme. One resident who grew up in Chicago might love a kit that has Chicago landmark postcards, a Cubs hat, a small toy sailboat, photos of pizza and hot dogs, and Chicago music. A wedding kit might include assorted silk flowers, a hankie, a piece of lace, a veil, photos of wedding cake, and wedding march music.

These objects are meant to be taken out and passed around one at a time. You use the object to kick off a discussion. For example, as you pass out the wedding hankie, you can ask if they cried at all during their wedding. Why did they cry? Did their dad walk them down the aisle? Were they excited to get married or nervous?

Ideally, your reminiscing kits will be multi-sensory and include a few different senses in each kit. While you cannot put food in the kit while you store it away in your resource closet, you could grab a food or drink item on your way to lead the group. For example, serve sparkling cider in plastic champagne flutes as part of your wedding discussion.

Discussion

What kind of tools do we have available in our community for reminiscence groups?

Lead one or two reminiscing groups with your participants, using the reminiscing kits and tools that you have available. Be sure that your staff know where your reminiscing kits and tools are located in your community so that they can easily access them next time they are leading a group.

Discussion

Are our current supplies working well in your groups and one-on-one interactions? Do we need to restock certain supplies?

Let's think of three new reminiscing kits, and the objects that will go in them, based on our current residents.

Remember, use open-ended phrases to start up a reminiscing conversation, instead of simple "yes or no" questions. For example, a question such as "Did you like your wedding dress?" will not trigger a set of memories. Instead, you might ask, "What did your wedding dress look like?" The latter question allows your resident(s) to give more detail and remember more about that special day.

Discussion

Let's brainstorm some good go-to topics for reminiscing. Examples might be wedding day, first and favorite cars, favorite things to do in the summertime, favorite foods or recipes, etc.

Inservice #11
Leading a Successful Reminiscence Group

Inservice Overview: Tips on how to lead a successful reminiscence group and why reminiscing is important to our residents
Presented by:________________________________
Date:________________________________
Start Time:________________________________
End Time:________________________________

NAME	DEPARTMENT

12.
Yearly Wrap Up

Staff training on federal, state, and community regulations, protocols, and procedures.

Topics
Yearly training done on back safety, resident rights, abuse and neglect, community's mission statement, severe weather and fire safety, confidentiality and privacy.

Who to Invite
Activity staff, CNA staff who lead programs with residents, volunteers.

Time
30-40 minutes.

Supplies
Inservice sign-in sheet.

Review Material
State and federal guidelines for your specific community.
Community-specific information.
Additional yearly training required by your community.
You can likely find all of this information and corresponding handouts in a new staff or volunteer orientation manual.

Content Reminders
This training covers general information that is reviewed on a yearly basis. The brief outline is a guide to be sure you have everything covered. Add other topics as required.
Use this opportunity to have a nurse come in and do yearly TB tests.

We will use this inservice to go over a set of important information related to our work. These yearly reminders help us keep this information in the forefront of our minds.

1. Resident Rights
2. Abuse and Neglect
3. Back Safety and Correct Lifting
4. Our Community's Mission Statement
5. Severe Weather and Fire Safety
6. Confidentiality and Privacy

Inservice #12
Yearly Wrap Up

Inservice Overview: Yearly training on back safety, resident rights, abuse and neglect, community's mission statement, severe weather and fire safety, confidentiality and privacy

Presented by:____

Date:____

Start Time:____

End Time:____

NAME	DEPARTMENT

13.
Spice Up Your Exercise

Adding variety to your exercise and other physical programming groups.

Topics
How to add variety to your exercise and other physical programming groups.

Who to Invite
Activity staff, CNA staff who lead programs with residents, volunteers who lead or assist with exercise programs, therapy staff.

Time
20 minutes, plus five minutes for each demonstration, plus time to brainstorm with other groups that attend.

Supplies
Inservice sign-in sheet.
Examples of exercise resources that you have at your community.

Review Material
Exercise programs (an exercise DVD or CD, Thera-bands, weights, hula-hoop, Christmas wreath, etc.).

Content Reminders
This training should be interactive, and you will ideally be leading the group in small "tastes" of the techniques described.
It will be a fun way for the participants to learn not only the technique, but to also see you model how to lead a group.
If you have other ideas, please add them to the training as well.

Exercise is an important part of our activity calendar and it is an important part of the lives and wellbeing of our residents. However, leading exercise can be a little tricky. We want our residents to get a nice range of motion workout, and we also want them to enjoy being there. Keeping exercise groups fresh, exciting, and drawing a crowd can be a difficult task sometimes. You might find yourself doing the exact same routine each time you lead exercise for the residents. This can be boring. And if you are bored, chances are high that your residents are bored, too.

Discussion

Do you like leading exercise and physical activity groups? Why or why not?

Do you sometimes feel that your exercise groups need something different to break the monotony?

Let's find a few ways to make exercise a little bit more exciting and engaging for our residents and for you!

Give it a Theme

If we are having a special day, week, or month here at the community, we should match our exercise to the theme. For example, during our beach month, we could do our exercise group to the music of the Beach Boys. Oktoberfest calls for polka music during exercise, and the entire month of December can feature Christmas carol exercise music.

Brainstorm some upcoming months and possible theme ideas that could be brought in to exercise programming.

Use Props

Now that we have themed music happening, let's add in some fun props. How about beach balls for each person during our Beach Boys exercise class, beer steins for Oktoberfest, and Christmas wreaths for December? We are only limited by our imaginations on how to use props. It gives residents something different to have in their hands and can add a little weight resistance, too. We could even title one exercise group per week "Prop-ercise" and have a different prop to use each time.

Now is a time to turn on a piece of music and demonstrate how to use themed music and props for exercise. Encourage everyone to participate and have some fun with it.

Use Some Help

If you are looking for something different, try using one of the exercise DVDs or CDs that we have available in the office. You can use parts or tracks of the DVD or CD, and it will be nice for someone else to do the leading. You will also be able to learn new exercises to add to your repertoire.

Demonstrate a DVD and CD here. Encourage everyone to participate.

Add Some Weight

If you are looking to spice up your exercise a bit, you can use some of the tools that we have here. You can use TheraBands, weights, or even cans of soup to add a bit of weight resistance. You are never too old to build muscle mass. When our residents gain strength, they will improve transfers and even increase independence.

Demonstrate a few new exercises with the weighted props you brought.

Leave the Circle

We don't need to use a circle for exercise. Exercise can look different to residents and it should look different on our calendar, too. Walking clubs, Wii games, yoga, and tai chi can and should be a part of what we offer to residents.

Brainstorm here as a group about what other types of physical activity you can offer besides exercise. Think about at least one offering you can add to next month's calendar.

Give Rewards and Incentives

Think about printing out exercise punch cards to pass out to residents. For each exercise group they attend, staff will punch their card. Once they fill a card full of punches, they get a prize — $5 to spend at the community store, a healthy snack pack, etc. You might be surprised when it gets different residents to attend your groups. Run the promotion for a month and then try it again a few months later. Don't forget to promote your punch card program in the newsletter and throughout your community in the elevators, dining room, etc.

Brainstorm this idea with the participants and come up with a target date to try it together.

Leave Them Guessing

Sometimes, the word "exercise" on our calendar turns off residents before we can even invite them. The word can have so many different connotations and meanings to people, including our residents. How about we consider changing the name and call it what it is. If it is a program based more on stretching, let's title it appropriately. If the group is made for beginners, let's say so. We can label something "Polkacise" or "Prop-ercise" and our group might increase just because some residents want to see exactly what is going to happen at the group.

Brainstorm ways to switch up some of the names of the exercise programs you offer.

Lead Fun and Good Groups

This might seem silly to even mention, but as long as you are running consistent, fun, and good quality exercise groups, your numbers will eventually grow. Residents who attended will be talking about it at lunch and during their coffee groups, encouraging others to check it out.

Discussion

What are some other ways that you make your exercise groups more exciting and engaging for the residents?

What are some challenges or obstacles that we have to making our exercise program extra special?

Pair Exercise with Therapy

Now let's look at one more idea for making our exercise program better than before. Our therapists can assist us in leading groups. It is a win-win for everyone. Therapists can count the group as a therapy session, as long as they meet appropriate resident-to-staff ratios. Residents get to see staff working together, you can learn a few different exercises, and it is nice to be able to have fun together. You can check with your restorative program as well and see if there is a possibility to run exercise together.

Have your therapy department staff brainstorm this idea with your activities staff. You can learn what the Medicare and Medicaid regulations say about co-treating and find a time when you can try it together.

Discussion

How can departments work together to increase resident participation in activities?

Is there anything specific that CNAs and nursing staff can do to help residents exercise in groups or on their own? Examples might be doing exercise and passive range of motion during morning or evening care, getting residents in proper exercise attire before groups, etc.

What are the action items for the next few months?

Inservice #13
Spice Up Your Exercise

Inservice Overview: How to add variety to your exercise and other physical programming groups

Presented by:____________________

Date:____________________

Start Time:____________________

End Time:____________________

NAME	DEPARTMENT

14.
Quality of Life

Description of the federal quality of life tag and making it come alive in the community.

Topics
Description of federal tag on quality of life and ways to make it come alive in the community.

Who to Invite
Activity staff, CNA staff who lead programs with residents, department managers, administrator.

Time
30-40 minutes.

Supplies
Inservice sign-in sheet.

Review Material
Community policies on quality of life.
Federal and state regulations on quality of life.
Tags F240-248 (with a special emphasis on F248) and the interpretive guidelines (483.15).

Content Reminders
Be familiar with the information.

In federal regulations, most activities fall under tag F248. Each tag has a set of interpretive guidelines that surveyors use to evaluate compliance with the tag. F248 is associated with other Quality of Life tags. This really is a good place for activities to be evaluated. Our activities should increase quality of life for our residents while they are here at our community.

F248 reads, "The facility must provide for an ongoing program of activities designed to meet, in accordance with the comprehensive assessment, the interests, and the physical, mental, and psychosocial well-being of each resident." This is not an easy requirement to evaluate. The interpretive guidelines are 13 pages long. The investigative protocol takes up another nine pages.

We are not going to read over all 22 pages of protocol and guidelines today. I do think that it is important for each of you to read all of them at least once a year. This would be on your own, as part of work. Please come by the office and I will show you where the guidelines are kept. Informed activity staff are the best activity staff!

The interesting thing about this tag is that it says all staff are responsible for providing activities. It does not say that the activity department is solely responsible. Everyone is responsible for knowing resident interests and preferences when it comes to recreation.

However, this does not mean that activity staff get to take it easy. I see us as the leaders. We are the experts in all things recreation for our residents. It is our responsibility to make our information and tools available to all of the staff in our community, not just to our department. Today, we are going to take a look at what that might look like. We'll find ways to lead the activities' quality of life program for our residents.

Discussion

How does resident choice and preference factor into our programming?

If a resident wants to participate in an independent leisure pursuit at midnight, as he or she has always been a night owl, is that okay? What is our role in making that happen?

While we are required to complete activity assessments and interest surveys on our residents, all our community staff are not required to read this information. We need to find out how to best communicate leisure interests to the staff here at our community.

The first place we should start is the care plan. The more thorough we are with interventions and information in our care plans, the better. Staff on all shifts are required to be up to date on care plans. Essentially, the care plan is a one-stop shop for resident information that is personalized and organized.

However, we should try to do more than just the care plan because we all know that things get busy. Staff might not be reading through the entire resident care plan, including activities. We need to make it easier. Could we make an activity preference half sheet and post it in each resident's closet? Could we have a binder with one page of activity information on each resident at the nursing station? Do we start attending crossover or shift-change meetings to pass along leisure information about residents? It might look different in our community, and we might have to try a few things before we figure it out, but it is important that we do.

Discussion

How do we currently pass along information about resident interests in programs?

How can we better communicate resident interests to other staff members?

What are two ways to pass along information that we will try together with the whole team over the next month?

In addition to informing other staff about resident interests, we also need to make activity supplies and independent leisure materials readily available and easily accessible for staff. Materials need to be accessible at all hours, even when we are not here. Materials also need to be based on current resident interests. For example, we might have a shelf full of cards and dominoes. However, if our residents are mostly interested in computers and books, we are not meeting that need. We are not giving all staff the tools to succeed.

Federal and state surveyors will expect that a resident who wants to read books at midnight can get books at midnight. Activity staff are typically not here at midnight. We need to be sure that the staff who are here during those hours know where to get the books for that resident. The same is true for anything else a resident might want.

What does that preparation look like for our community? Do we keep a small box of supplies based on resident interest in each resident's nightstand? Do we keep a shelf of materials at each nursing station?

And, what about instructions on how to use the materials? If we have a reminiscing kit available for Mr. Jones, the staff might not know how to use it with him.

Discussion

How can we have accessible materials and instructions at our community?

How can we communicate how to best use our tools and the directions for games or other materials?

What are two ways to make materials available that we will try together with the whole team over the next month?

One of the best ways that we can encourage staff participation in activities and overall quality of life for our residents is to be good models of the behavior. Lead your groups with excitement and invite staff to attend groups, too. If you see staff peeking in on your event, ask them to come in. If you find a leisure intervention that works well with a resident, tell the nursing staff and show them where the materials are kept. Also, if a staff member tells you something that works with a resident, take that information to heart and thank them for passing it along. The more we all communicate with one another about resident needs and preferences, the better we are serving our residents.

Discussion

How can we be good role models for leading and providing activities for residents?

How can we encourage staff to become more involved with us?

How can staff from each department tell us about resident preferences and reactions to activities?

One group that sometimes gets left out of the quality of life process is the resident's family. We need to find ways to bring the families into the process, too.

Discussion

How can we work with resident families to involve them in the resident's pursuit of better quality of life?

Do family members feel a part of the life of our community here? How can we make this happen?

Inservice #14
Quality of Life

Inservice Overview: Description of federal tag on quality of life and ways to make it come alive in the community

Presented by:____________________

Date:____________________

Start Time:____________________

End Time:____________________

NAME	DEPARTMENT

15.
Dining and Activities

Incorporate food into activities in a fun and safe way. Working with the dining team.

Topics
How to incorporate food into activities in a fun and safe way. Working with the dining team to make it easy on everyone.

Who to Invite
Activity staff, CNA staff who lead programs with residents, volunteers who lead or assist with programs that involve food, dining staff.

Time
30-40 minutes.

Supplies
Inservice sign-in sheet.

Co-presenters
Director of dining services or another member of the dining staff.

Review Material
Food-specific information, guidelines, and safety precautions for your community.
Federal and state regulations related to food.

Content Reminders
The goal of this inservice is to foster an understanding of the roles of both dining and activities during the planning and implementation of activities for the residents. While some best practices and ideas are listed below, if those ideas are not pertinent to your community, please use your own examples.

Food and parties go hand in hand, no matter what age you are. In order to have a successful program that reaches many residents, dining and activities must work together to best serve our residents. Usually, activity staff and dining staff are creative people. When you get the two disciplines together and the brainstorming starts, you can get some amazing and fun results that benefit the whole community.

Discussion

How do our activity and dining teams work together here at our community?

I think that we will all agree that while having a party with beautiful decorations and entertainment is great, the event becomes even better with food. We must work together to plan and execute dining service during some of our events to make them extra special. But before we can start talking about what food to serve, we first have to talk about how to safely serve the food.

Discussion

Use this time to review food safety and food service guidelines from your local health department as well as federal and state regulations. The dining director might be the best person to present this information. Be sure you are offering practical information to your activity staff: Do they need to wear gloves or hairnets? When do they wash their hands and how often? Leave time for attendees to ask questions.

Now that we have safe food service covered, we can start to think about what kind of food works best with different events. Let's take a moment to touch on specialized diets and options we have available for our residents with special needs.

Discussion

Cover your community policy on specialized diets. Some communities offer a more liberal approach when it comes to special diets and activities, while others do not. Cover special diets like diabetic diets, no added salt diets, and weight-loss or weight-gain diets, in addition to mechanical soft and pureed diets. Now is also a good time to cover who is allowed to feed residents who might require assistance, based on your community and state regulations.

When we think about what to serve at events, we need to consider how easy it is to serve and how easy it is to eat. Serving caramel apples, for example, might fit a fall social beautifully. Unfortunately, it is not very realistic for our residents. Most of them have dentures that make caramel apples hard to bite into and enjoy. Sliced apples with a caramel dipping sauce might be a better idea. Similarly, having a choose-your-own ice cream sundae bar with 20 topping choices and 40 residents in attendance would be a nightmare if there is only one activity staff to serve them.

Besides ease of service and ease of eating, we must consider the timing of events where we serve food. Having a pie-tasting social might not be the best idea immediately following lunch. Residents will be full and participation might decrease. Having the pie-tasting social too close to the beginning of dinner might not work either. However, having the same pie-tasting social might be perfect in the middle of the afternoon, around 3 p.m. It gives time for residents to digest their lunch, and it doesn't ruin their dinner appetite. Sometimes, timing is everything.

Once we have our timing down, we can decide what we want to serve. Having a cinnamon roll social in the evening is not as good as having the same social in the midmorning. A happy hour that serves cheese, crackers, and fruit is the perfect idea for an event right before dinner in the dining room. Donuts and coffee is a perfect menu for a Saturday morning current events group. Cookies and hot tea might serve a Saturday afternoon current events gathering.

Discussion

What kinds of events do we serve food at?

How is that going: for dining staff, for activities staff, and for the residents? What can we improve on? What do we do well?

What is the current role of volunteers with dining during activities? How can we get the volunteers more involved in helping dining with serving and setting up our events?

We want to strive to be sure our residents don't become bored with our food offerings. This is where our creativity comes in. While we want to keep resident favorites in our rotation of food served at events, we want to keep it interesting as well. Finding a food choice that matches our event theme is usually the best way to keep our menu exciting. A beach themed party can offer fruit kabobs. A Chinese New Year celebration can offer crab Rangoon or egg rolls. We want to keep a good balance of healthy to decadent food. That means we can't serve brownies at each event.

And let's not forget drinks! We don't always have to serve food at events to add to the festivities. Sometimes, a drink is all it takes. Adding drinks besides coffee and water to events is an easy way to make the event seem a little more special. We can call a fizzing pink punch "Love Potion Number 9." That can be served while watching *Casablanca* during our Valentine's Day celebrations. Hot chocolate can become a "Ho Ho Ho Hot Cocoa" during Christmas events. Make it extra special by adding whipped cream and a mini candy cane to the cup!

Discussion

How do you think we are doing on our food choices at events? What can we do better?

As a team, let's pick a few upcoming events and plan for the food and drink choices.

Inservice #15
Dining and Activities

Inservice Overview: How to incorporate food into activities in a fun and safe way. Working with the dining team to make it easy on everyone

Presented by:______________________________

Date:______________________________

Start Time:______________________________

End Time:______________________________

NAME	DEPARTMENT

16.
Working with Therapy

How activities and therapy can work hand in hand.

Topics
Tips and examples of how activities and therapy can work hand in hand for outstanding results.

Who to Invite
Activity staff, CNA staff who lead programs with residents, therapy staff.

Time
30-40 minutes.

Supplies
Inservice sign-in sheet.

Co-presenters
Director of therapy services or a member of the therapy staff.

Review Material
Information and guidelines specific to your community.
Policies.
Federal and state regulations.
CMS guidelines.

Content Reminders
Allow the class to be the start of an honest conversation about how the two departments work together in your community and a brainstorming session on how you can best work together to serve the residents.

We have an amazing chance to make our residents' lives better by working with our physical therapy, occupational therapy, and speech therapy team members. We can pair the rehabilitation and restorative side of their job with the social and emotional part of our job. This lets residents have a variety of dimensions of wellness in one program or event.

It can be difficult to foster that connection between activities and therapy, though. While it might not be true here, other communities struggle with the therapy-activities partnership. Activity staff may think that therapy steals their residents from programs. Therapy staff may think that activity staff do not respect the treatment times that the therapists must adhere to. There might be a little truth in both of these schools of thought. The better path is to work together. Then we can increase our resident satisfaction. We can help our residents get stronger together and give them confidence to go home independently.

There are a variety of ways that activities can partner with therapy. Before we hear some ideas and start making action steps for our community, let's be sure that we all understand what each group does.

Discussion

Have a member of activities describe, in one sentence, what activities does for the residents.

Do the same with members from the therapy side. There should be one each from physical, occupational, speech, and restorative. You can provide the information, if required.

Allow the other participants to ask questions about the departments.

Keep comments positive and curious.

Now that we have an idea of what we all do, and how we view the resident, let's look at some ways we can work together. While not all of these ideas will work for our community, we can get a good start by listening to these best practices.

One of the best places that therapy and activities can partner is on outings. Many residents need to work on certain goals or strength exercises. There is no better place to work on real-world needs than in the real world. At least monthly, if not more often, we can do therapy-specific trips. Activity staff and therapy staff meet to pick the destination and discuss which residents should be invited. Therapists attend the outing and assist as needed with transfers and with other actions that meet therapy goals. Activity staff run the outing and encourage socialization. The residents have a fun trip that gets them out of the therapy gym. Therapists can bill for the services as long as the therapist-to-resident ratio meets guidelines. It is also nice for the therapists to work with residents in a different setting. This type of trip can also work for our long-term residents who are on programs to build or restore strength. In this case, restorative therapists or CNA staff can attend the trip.

Activities can also work with therapy. A therapist and an activity staff can co-lead exercise groups, walking clubs, or any physical activity group. Activities can count the participants in their records. Therapists can bill for the group therapy session as long as the therapist-to-resident ratio meets guidelines. Therapists can provide a specific list of residents that activities can invite and gather. We can invite other residents as well, not just those on the therapy list. It is fun to have an exercise group led by two different people from two different disciplines. We can each learn from one another. It keeps the group engaging and exciting for our residents.

Most importantly, activities and therapy must communicate well. Therapists can post the day's therapy schedule in each resident's room. This helps the activity department when they are inviting and gathering residents for activities. Similarly, the activity department should provide a current event calendar for the therapy room. Therapists can ask residents as they leave the gym where they want to go. The residents might like to go back to their room. But they also might like to attend an activity when they are reminded of it. If a therapist is working with a resident who has memory issues and sees that activities is offering a Mind Games group, the therapist can encourage the resident to attend the group as a complement to the current therapy.

Discussion

How do activities staff currently communicate their activities to therapy?

How do therapy staff currently communicate their therapy times to activities?

How do we work together currently?

Are there any conflicts, scheduling or otherwise, that you have noticed? How can we address those conflicts together as a team that is focused on serving our residents?

What are some ways that we could improve our therapy-activities teamwork to best serve the residents?

Residents in our community have the right to choice. Both the therapy department and the activity department must recognize and respect this.

Discussion

Take a moment to review the resident's right to choose.

If a resident has been looking forward to a specific event for a week, we hope that the therapy team recognizes this and trades therapy times to avoid conflict with the special event. Similarly, if a resident is attending an activity group and elects to leave the group to attend therapy, the activity staff need to respect and honor the resident's choice.

Discussion

Let's brainstorm ideas on how to best work together. We won't leave here until we think of at least three things that we can try over the next month.

Inservice #16
Working with Therapy

Inservice Overview: Tips and examples of how activities and therapy can work hand in hand for outstanding results

Presented by:________________________________

Date:________________________________

Start Time:________________________________

End Time:________________________________

NAME	DEPARTMENT

17.
Reaching Residents Where They Are

Connecting with residents outside of groups.

Topics
Practical ideas on how to connect with residents in a variety of settings — the dining room, their room, in the hallway, before meals, etc. — not just in groups.

Who to Invite
Activity staff, CNA staff who lead programs with residents.

Time
30-40 minutes.

Supplies
Inservice sign-in sheet.

Content Reminders
This training should be informative and should also be a way to brainstorm program ideas together as a team. Be open to the ideas that the team comes up with and develop at least three workable ideas that you can use over the next month.

Let's think about our current activity calendar and the activities that you lead on a regular basis. How many of those activities are groups? Probably almost all of them. Most activity departments are group focused. It is okay to be group focused. The socialization and peer encouragement of group programming cannot be duplicated in one-on-one interactions.

However, what do we do when residents are not interested in groups? Or, what do we do when residents are only free from therapy, medical care, or resting during times when we do not have groups planned? Both of these situations are real. To be sure that residents are not slipping through the cracks, we need interventions that reach residents where they are.

Discussion

Do all of our residents like group activities?

Can you think of at least three current residents who never attend groups?

Why wouldn't residents want to attend groups?

What can we do besides groups and scheduled one-on-ones? Here are some ideas to get us started. Then I want us to spend a majority of this session brainstorming. We will work together to develop a plan for leading our groups and scheduled one-on-ones and still meet residents in other settings.

Stop-in Visits

It is a good goal for us to greet and do a stop-in visit for each of our residents every day that we work. A stop-in visit is typically not charted. It is just a chance to say hi to the resident. We get to see how they are feeling, give them a rundown of interesting activities for the day, and chat for a bit. Although these visits last less than five minutes each, they accomplish a lot. A stop-in visit tells the resident there are activities happening that day and puts a face to our activities department. Even if you feel like a resident does not like you stopping in to say hello, it might mean more to them than you realize.

Independent Leisure Cart

There is a more advanced stop-in visit that we could do here at our community a few times a week. This visit includes an independent leisure cart. We take it to each resident's room and offer something from the cart. Items on the cart promote independent leisure pursuits and could be charted. Ideas for things on the cart include crossword or sudoku puzzles, word searches, electronic games (labeled as property of the activities department), packs of playing cards, current magazines, current books from the library, CD players and CDs, paper notepads and sketchpads, and writing utensils. Residents who do not prefer groups, or who have a schedule or medical care that does not allow for group participation, might really enjoy the opportunity of the independent leisure cart.

Hydration Station

While we are talking about carts, let's consider partnering with dining and offering a fun twist on hydration. A few times a week, a member of our staff could take around a smoothie cart full of freshly made smoothies, fresh fruit, or fruit-infused water. We could pass out the goodies and use the time to remind residents of upcoming events or to check in on their supply of leisure materials.

Before-Meals Trivia

In most communities, a line begins to form 20 minutes before the dining room opens. That means that three times a day we have a captive audience who gathered themselves. Why aren't we taking advantage of this? We can grab a trivia book and some fun dollar-store prizes and head on over to the dining room a half-hour before meals to turn waiting into a fun activity.

Before-Dinner Happy Hour

Along the same lines, we can consider having a happy hour event near the dining room 30 minutes before dinner a few times per month. We could supply a cheese and cracker tray and a unique drink. Sometimes we might add a musician playing violin or piano. Then the before-dinner wait will be much more fun for everyone involved.

Town Crier

Before residents start to leave the dining room after eating, we have an opportunity to promote the day's activities. We can do this at breakfast or at lunch here in our community. It gives us the chance to swing into the dining room, sing a song, or talk a bit about current events before reminding residents of the activities for the day. If it is appropriate, we can end with a prayer, or we can offer some words of encouragement.

Discussion

Would any of these ideas work for our community? Why or why not?

How can we meet residents in non-group settings in order to promote our department and remind them of upcoming opportunities? Let's brainstorm and choose at least three ideas to develop into programs for the next month.

Inservice #17
Reaching Residents Where They Are

Inservice Overview: Practical ideas on how to connect with residents in a variety of settings — the dining room, their room, in the hallway, before meals, etc. — not just in groups.

Presented by:____

Date:____

Start Time:____

End Time:____

NAME	DEPARTMENT

18.
Working with the Family

Getting the family involved and active in events.

Topics
Why to get family involved and how to get them involved and active in events.

Who to Invite
Activity staff, CNA staff who lead programs with residents, marketing department staff.

Time
30-40 minutes.

Supplies
Inservice sign-in sheet.
Copies of current month's activity calendar.

Co-presenters
Director of marketing or other member of the community relations team, if you have a good working relationship with one another and work well together on family nights or other family events.

Review Material
Information and guidelines specific to your community.
State regulations regarding family involvement and Family Councils.

Content Reminders
Use lots of resident-specific examples and discussion to make this training even more meaningful.

For better or, sometimes, for worse, our residents' families are part of our everyday interactions here. Some family members are here on a daily basis. Some family members we never see, but it is a safe bet that many residents have family members or close friends that are invested in their care.

Discussion

How often do you interact with the family members of our residents?

In your opinion, what is our role in activities as it relates to family members?

Take a moment to think about a time when a loved one or close friend was in a hospital or medical setting. Chances are you were listening to the doctors and nurses just as much as the patient was. You were likely asking good questions and monitoring the care your loved one was receiving. This is also the case for our residents' family members. Once we see that these family members are a major part of the resident's life and plan of care, we can work with them to get them involved with events throughout our community.

While our number-one priority and our number-one customer is always the resident, we want family members to feel welcome as well. They will, after all, be spending quite a few hours, days, weeks, and months here at our community. We want them to see that we are providing excellent programming options for their loved one. It is our responsibility to educate both family members and the resident about the activities program. In many cases, the family members may be our strongest allies by providing extra encouragement for residents to participate in groups.

Best practices for educating family members include emailed and printed newsletters and calendars. The family members can also be part of, or even host, a monthly social to welcome new families. Include the administrator, director of nursing or assistant director of nursing, department heads, and therapy staff. Serve a light snack and have each department present a brief, no more than five-minute, introduction about their department. This is a relaxed way for family members to meet the care team.

Invite family members to attend groups with their loved one. This will let the family members see what we do in our groups and how their loved ones participate. Further, having family members attend events and programs can often persuade the resident to attend, too.

Discussion

How do we currently educate family members on the activity department and our programs?

What are some ways that we can do this better?

Do our resident family members receive a copy of our calendar via email or mail?

How can our volunteers help us in facilitating that communication about what activities we offer to our residents?

Having a Family Council is another way to get family members involved. This council does not have to be formal. It can meet monthly or quarterly.

Discussion

Let's discuss our current Family Council.

OR

Let's brainstorm if you think it would be a good idea to start a Family Council in our community.

Family nights allow the opportunity for family members and loved ones to have some fun together, and with the staff. Best practices typically call for monthly or quarterly family nights where all or most department heads stay to assist in the event. The focus for a family night should be on having fun and creating good memories with one another, so the theme should be light. Themes can include "An Evening at the Beach," "A Night at the Movies," or a holiday-themed event. Marketing should be involved in co-planning the event. There should be light refreshments, entertainment, and an activity for everyone to enjoy. Usually family nights should be after the dinner hour or at least after 5 p.m. so that family members who work can attend.

Discussion

Let's discuss our current family night plans at our community.

OR

We don't have a family night scheduled, let's brainstorm one now.

Brainstorm how you will get the word out to family members, residents, and staff.

Family nights aren't the only way to get families involved. Family members can be part of our regular activities, too. Let's take a look at our current activity calendar that you have in front of you now.

Discussion

What are some events that we could easily turn into a family-centered event by inviting family members and serving a snack?

What are some events that we could highlight in our upcoming newsletter with an invitation for families to stop by and check them out?

Working with families can be beneficial for everyone involved. Let's think of specific ways we can invite them to be part of our community.

Discussion

What is one thing that you will do over the next month to connect more with families?

What is one thing that our department can focus on over the next month to increase family communication?

Should we highlight activities on our calendar or newsletter that families are encouraged to participate in? Or would this discourage families from attending other activities?

Inservice #18
Working with the Family

Inservice Overview: Why to get family involved, how to get them involved and active in events
Presented by:______________________________
Date:______________________________
Start Time:______________________________
End Time:______________________________

NAME	DEPARTMENT

19. Spiritual Life

Spiritual and religious practices in the community.

Topics
Introduction to the importance of spiritual and religious practices in the lives of residents. How to implement them in a meaningful way at the community.

Who to Invite
Activity staff, CNA staff who lead programs with residents, volunteers who lead spiritual-based programs, chaplain.

Time
30-40 minutes.

Supplies
Inservice sign-in sheet.

Co-presenters
Chaplain.

Review Material
Community policies on spiritual life.
State and federal regulations about spiritual and religious pursuit.

Content Reminders
Pull residents' interest sheets to get spiritual information to use during the training. Use lots of resident-specific examples and discussion to make this training even more meaningful.

When you hear the word "spiritual," do you automatically think of religion, God, the devil, and heaven? It is okay if you do make that instant connection, but it is also okay if you see "spiritual" and "religion" as two completely different things. I bet our some of our residents make that connection and some do not. That is okay, too. But I do think it is important that we all agree on one thing — spiritual programming has an important place here at our community.

Discussion

What do you think about as part of spiritual life?

Let's start by looking at the state and federal regulations related to spiritual practice.

Review your state-specific regulatory guidelines about spiritual/religious programming.

Beyond the regulations, we want to offer spiritual programming to our residents because it is an important part of complete wellness. When we learned about the dimensions of wellness, if you remember, spiritual life was one of them. What makes spiritual and religious programming a little tricky is that some of us were taught to never talk about religion, especially at work. However, our role here in our community requires us to be able to talk about spiritual and religious programming needs and interests, just as much as the card game preferences of our residents.

Many of our residents want to be involved in spiritual or religious programming. Let's take a look at some of the interest sheets we have for residents.

Discussion

What kind of spiritual involvement and preferences can we find in the residents currently in our community?

How many are Catholic? Protestant? Jewish? Hindu? Muslim? Other faiths?

Substitute examples from your community that show an easily satisfied resident and a resident who is harder to program for.

Let's start by talking organized religion. Sometimes, it is easy for us to meet the religious needs of our residents. For example, Mrs. Anderson is Catholic. We have rosary happening in our activity room once a week. We can invite her to that. There is also a mass held here in our community on the first Sunday of the month. Participating in these events might meet Mrs. Anderson's religious needs quite well.

Sometimes it can be a bit harder, especially if we do not have programs already in place or resources readily available. Mrs. Goldring is Jewish. Even though we don't have a temple close to our community, it is still our responsibility to meet her needs. We need to find a rabbi to visit and find a Torah to give to her to use. If she chooses, we must respect her preference to celebrate the traditional Jewish Sabbath beginning on Friday night at sundown.

It doesn't matter what organized religion is important to each of our residents. It is our responsibility to offer them a way to feel connected to that religion and higher power.

Spirituality, on the other hand, can be different. I have had residents say, "I'm not religious, but I am spiritual." This statement shows that while this resident might not be interested in organized church services, he or she still desires a way to feel connected to something other than himself or herself. Spiritual programming that we can offer here might include gardening, yoga or tai chi, meditation, prayer groups, labyrinth walking, deep breathing groups, or even guided imagery. However, the best way to find out how a person connects to things spiritually is to ask that person. Former athletes might connect spiritually by running. In that case, could we get him or her involved with planning our exercise groups? Former teachers might connect spiritually by interacting with children. Could we invite that resident to our next intergenerational program?

Discussion

How do you think we are doing now with meeting the religious and spiritual needs of our residents?

How could we get better at meeting these needs?

Can you think of a current resident who needs a religious or spiritual program or resource that we are not providing?

Let's brainstorm together and find ways to best meet that need.

Some of our residents have recently faced, or are currently facing, a major medical crisis. Some of our residents are facing end-of-life decisions or end-of-life care. In cases such as these, friendly and compassionate listening can do wonders for their mood and spirituality. You might hear a resident ask for a Bible or for prayer when you have never heard that resident previously express an interest in religion or spiritual care. You might see a resident's family member sobbing in the hallway, or praying out loud in our chapel. When you sense a greater religious or spiritual need, do you know what to do?

Talk about your chaplain services for residents and for family members. If your community does not have a chaplain, talk about social services or a visiting pastor or religious leader who is available to residents and family members.

Discussion

How can we use these services with our residents and families?

Inservice #19
Spiritual Life

Inservice Overview: The importance of spiritual and religious practices in the lives of residents and how to implement them in a meaningful way at the community

Presented by:____

Date:____

Start Time:____

End Time:____

NAME	DEPARTMENT

20.
Grieving and Letting Go

Dealing with our residents' losses and our losses in a healthy way.

Topics
Information focused on losses that our residents may be experiencing, losses that we experience while working with seniors, and how to deal with them in appropriate and healthy ways.

Who to Invite
Activity staff, CNA staff, nursing staff, social services staff.

Time
50-60 minutes.

Supplies
Inservice sign-in sheet.
Paper and pens for everyone in the class.

Co-presenters
Social services director or chaplain.

Content Reminders
Use lots of resident-specific examples, staff examples, and discussion for even more meaning.

Loss is something that we all experience. At least once, you have likely experienced a loss that shook you to the core. You have likely grieved for someone or something in your lifetime, and the older we get, the more losses we experience. In our time together today, we are going to talk about losses that our residents experience, losses that we might experience while working here, and healthy ways to cope.

Activity

To start us off, let's do a quick activity. Everyone should have a piece of paper and pen. I would like you to tear your paper so that you have eight small pieces. On each of those small pieces of paper, write down one thing that is very important to you. When you are done, you will have eight pieces of paper with eight different things written on them.

Once everyone is done writing, pick one sheet of paper, look at the thing on the paper, and crumble it up. Pretend that you have lost the thing that was on the paper and you no longer have it.

Do this with each of the eight items you have. Crumple them up and pretend those items are gone from your life, never to return.

How does it feel to lose items or people from your life?

What kinds of losses are our residents experiencing when they come to us or while they are here?

Because we strive to be resident-centered, let's start by focusing on our residents and the losses that they have had or will have while under our care. Losses our residents have faced, currently face, or will face are varied and include people, relationships, abilities, and physical things. We must grasp these losses and what they mean to our residents in order for us to respect the severity of the losses that our residents experience.

Our residents have lost, and are grieving for, people important to them. As we age, we die. This is a fact. However, it certainly does not make losing someone any easier. Our residents might have lost a spouse, friends, siblings, children, grandchildren, mentors, or business partners. Imagine your best friend right now and think about how long you have known him or her. Now, imagine being best friends with that same person until you are 90 — you could be looking at 80 years of friendship with the same person. That is a long time, full of rich memories, sharing, and love. When our residents lose these important people, they are not only grieving the loss of that particular person, but also what that person meant to the resident and the memories they shared. The resident is grieving how his or her life will now be drastically different from what it was before, when that person was alive.

Our residents may have lost relationships. I am sure that all of you can respect the fact that relationships in our lives are complicated and ever-changing. This holds true with our residents, and many times the older we get, the more complicated those relationships get. Medical crises and scary diagnoses can make families fall apart. It is likely that we have all seen that during our time working with seniors. Our residents might be grieving a relationship that we know nothing about, yet that relationship might not be broken or damaged, though sometimes it is. A daughter and grandchildren that live far away or a son that doesn't visit as often as our resident would like can all be cause for grieving.

Our residents are grieving their own bodies and physical limitations. This is a big one that we often overlook or try to sugarcoat. However, it is a very real loss for our residents. Imagine not being able to go to the bathroom without assistance or not being able to knit or button your blouse due to crippling arthritis. Our residents are grieving the ability to hear or see the way they once did and grieving a body that was once able to move faster and without as much aching as it does now. Losing memory or feeling like your body is betraying you requires grieving before our residents can emotionally move one.

Finally, our residents are losing real, physical items. Our residents have lost the family home that they lived in, raised their children in, and created memories in. They have lost their car. They have perhaps lost control of their money, or have watched as many of their possessions were sold. They may now only have the possessions that are in their small room. We must realize that these items signify more than just things. They also represent memories, independence, and control.

Discussion

What are some other things that our residents have lost?

Working with seniors means that we are more susceptible to losing things, too. Chances are, if you work here, you are already a compassionate person. You are probably the one in your family that everyone comes to when they need help. You always want to help. You wear your heart on your sleeve. You are a caregiver by nature. You love people. You love our residents and the relationships that you form with them. If this doesn't describe you at least a little bit, perhaps you are in the wrong profession.

We are all caregivers, helpers, givers. This innate compassion that we all have, along with our desire to help those who are aging, can lead to some loss in our own work lives that we need to be able to recognize and respect.

As caregivers, we lose people. Our residents age, our residents die. This reality is hard, but true. While you work here or in any health care setting, you will experience the loss of a "favorite" resident, the shocking loss of a very active resident who died suddenly, or the long and drawn-out death of a hospice resident. It will hurt every time. Still, we need to cope with these losses in a healthy way so that we do not stop ourselves from building relationships with other residents in the hopes of avoiding another hurt.

Discussion

What losses have you experienced since working in a health care setting?

Can you share about a time when a resident's death hit you particularly hard?

As caregivers, we run the risk of losing ourselves. If we give and give and give to other people, but do not take time to give back to ourselves, we will burn out. There is nothing worse than seeing coworkers burn out and eventually quit or hate their job because they are working too many hours and giving too much of themselves away without refueling. You must learn how to cope and have a healthy balance of work and personal life so that you can give all you can while you are at work, but also have the self-awareness to know what you need to do during off-hours to recharge your batteries.

Coping with loss and grieving is a conscious effort. We must find healthy ways to cope with losses that we experience here at work, and we must encourage our residents to find healthy ways to cope with the losses that they are experiencing as well. While your way of healthy coping might not look the same as mine, we can learn a variety of different techniques and use ones that fit our preferences and personality. Here are a few ideas to get us started.

Grieve. Recognize that you have experienced a loss and know that it is okay to grieve. There is no right or wrong way to grieve. You will experience many emotions during the grieving process. Give yourself permission to grieve and be gentle with yourself when you have a bad day.

Create. Whether you choose to write in a journal, draw or sketch, paint, garden, or dance, creating something can be a healthy outlet for stress caused by loss or grief. Making something new and beautiful is a wonderful antidote for a loss.

Get physical. Burn off stress and get a shot of natural endorphins by exercising. Whether you choose to run, walk, Zumba, do yoga, bike, or another type of exercise, as long as you are moving, you are helping yourself stay healthy and getting a natural "feel-good high" to help carry you through your loss.

Know your limits. When you are feeling burned out, you must be honest with yourself, your family, and your supervisor. If you know that you emotionally cannot work another 12-hour shift, say so. Also, be responsible to yourself and your family by taking your vacation days. You need time to recharge and refresh yourself. Your vacation days are an ideal time for you to focus on yourself and what really matters to you, outside of work.

Talk it out. Whether you talk to a trusted co-worker, family member, or therapist, you need an outlet to talk about your bad days, your hard days, and your good days.

Discussion

How do you cope with loss that you experience here at work?

What are some healthy coping skills that work for you that you can share?

Inservice #20
Grieving and Letting Go

Inservice Overview: Losses that our residents may be experiencing, losses that we experience while working with seniors, and how to deal with them in an appropriate and healthy way

Presented by:______________________________

Date:______________________________

Start Time:______________________________

End Time:______________________________

NAME	DEPARTMENT

21.
Activity's Role in Discharge

The role of the activities department in discharge planning and preparation.

Topics
Importance of activity's role in resident discharge planning and community resources for our discharged residents.

Who to Invite
Activity staff, CNA staff who lead activity programs, care plan coordinator, social services staff, discharge coordinator, department managers.

Time
30-40 minutes.

Supplies
Inservice sign-in sheet.
Brochures of community resources such as park district program guides, local senior center program guides, local theater brochures, local bowling alley brochures, etc.

Co-presenters
Social worker.
Discharge coordinator.

Review Material
Community-specific discharge tools.
State-specific regulations on discharge.

Content Reminders
Be prepared with information about the discharge process when you lead this training.

When our residents first enter our community, whether from home or from the hospital, they usually do not know what to expect when it comes to their care, the food, or the activities. Often, as a resident starts feeling better and has pain under control, and as he or she gets into the swing of our routine here, we start to notice that participation in our programs increases. Sometimes, we are taken by surprise. We might think that a certain resident would never get involved with our programs and now he or she comes to everything that we do. I love when this happens! But there is something to be said about living in a community like ours. It is different than living at home, alone.

In many ways, living in a community setting is better than living at home, especially for social interaction. There is always someone to talk to here, at all hours of the day and night. There is almost always something going on for a resident who is bored or wanting to get out of the room. And leisure materials are always available for resident use. At home, especially if a resident lives alone, chances are high that a majority of the time is spent in a recliner or couch, watching television or doing another type of sedentary and isolated activity. Now, that is not to say that scenario is happening everywhere. We have seen plenty of very active residents who live at home alone and who are hardly ever at home or alone! But, unfortunately, if a resident lives alone with little social support, the active lifestyle he or she might foster here in our community will evaporate.

Discussion

Can you think of a resident that is very active here at our community, but who has a sedentary and isolated lifestyle at home? Share that with the group.

Is it important that residents remain active — socially, physically, and intellectually — when they return home? Why or why not?

We can encourage our residents to remain socially fit once they return home as long as we get actively involved with their discharge.

Discussion

How are we active in a resident's discharge right now?

Do you think that is enough or could we be doing more?

Let's review the discharge process.

Discussion

Review the process at your specific community. You can review the discharge timeline or you can ask your social worker or discharge coordinator to review it for the group. Include items such as:

Who decides that a resident is getting close to discharge?

On average, how many days before discharge do we know about it?

When a resident is approaching discharge, is there a discharge planning meeting? If so, who attends this meeting?

How is the activity department currently involved with discharge?

What types of materials does a discharged resident go home with? Medication, prescriptions, doctor notes, follow-up appointments, etc.

After discharge, do we follow up with residents at home via phone calls within a set time frame?

When residents go home, I think that it is fair to say that they are likely experiencing a variety of emotions. While happy to be returning home, there are often issues. Some might experience anxiety or worry about safety. Some might lack confidence in themselves. Some might be overwhelmed with wondering how they will get to and from therapy and doctor appointments. Some might be embarrassed or sad about their current medical condition and how much they have changed since their medical crisis.

I believe that if we make an effort to get involved with resident discharge, we can make a positive impact on their emotional state when they return home. I want us to share ideas and brainstorm together on how we could get involved with discharge planning more. But first, here are a few best practices that we could learn from, and even consider adapting to fit our community.

Talk about It

When we know about an upcoming discharge, all members of the activity department can talk about it with the resident as it comes up. The more residents are able to talk openly about their discharge as well as any emotions that come along with it, the better they can handle it. I think we would all agree that residents have a different relationship with the activity department. So, we must not be surprised by an upcoming discharge if we want to allow the resident the opportunity to talk it through.

Strategize

We want our residents to be involved and socially connected here at our community as well as when they return home. Once we know about an upcoming discharge, we can strategize as a team that includes the resident to develop a plan and resources so that the resident can remain active at home. If we know that a resident loves our exercise class and attends daily, let's work with her to find a Silver Sneakers or other senior exercise class that is close to her home. We'll need to know our greater community resources for this, and we'll talk more about that in just a moment. But, first, we cannot underestimate the power of developing an easy-to-follow plan for our residents. We want the plan to be failure-free so that the resident feels comfortable and confident that it can be accomplished. We also want the resident to feel excited about it!

Know the Greater Community

We should be well connected with our local senior centers, park districts, and home health companies. A best practice is for the activity department to have a binder full of activity resources for the greater community like a current park district programming guide, the current senior center newsletter, a listing of free classes for seniors offered by therapy and home health companies, etc.

Work with Other Departments

There is no reason to reinvent the wheel, and no reason for us to feel like we have to step out of our specialty to meet the social discharge needs of our residents. If you and the resident find an exercise class to attend once discharged, but the resident is not sure how to get there, let's work with the social work or discharge department to find contacts for local transportation companies or family connections.

Discussion

How do we make sure we know about upcoming discharges?

Let's brainstorm together and think about how we could become more involved with resident discharge. We'll develop a list of all the ideas and then, as a team, let's choose two to focus on first.

Inservice #21
Our Role in Discharge

Inservice Overview: Importance of activity's role in resident discharge planning, and community resources for our discharged residents

Presented by:________________________________

Date:________________________________

Start Time:________________________________

End Time:________________________________

NAME	DEPARTMENT

22.
Depression and Anxiety

The effect of depression and anxiety on participation in leisure activities.

Topics
Information about depression and anxiety, and how it might affect participation in programs.

Who to Invite
Activity staff, CNA staff who lead activity programs, social services staff, care plan coordinator.

Time
30-40 minutes.

Supplies
Inservice sign-in sheet.

Co-presenters
Social services director.

Review Material
Latest information on depression and anxiety from the National Alliance on Mental Illness and other sources.

Content Reminders
Provide examples using current residents, when possible.

We often see depression and anxiety diagnoses when we work with seniors. According to the National Alliance on Mental Illness (NAMI), depression affects more than 6.5 million adults over the age of 65. The American Psychological Association (APA) estimates that as many as 37% of seniors in primary care settings suffer from depression. About 11% of seniors over the age of 65 have an anxiety disorder. Many of the seniors we serve are diagnosed with one or the other, or both. Both NAMI and the APA also estimate that these numbers are low. There are probably many seniors who are suffering with either depression or anxiety but are not diagnosed.

Some seniors have had a depression diagnosis before in their life. Others never suffered from depression until their senior years. A variety of factors can contribute to an onset of depression in later years of life. These include isolation and loneliness, grief about loss, physical ailments, and health issues.

Anxiety disorders are similar. Some seniors have struggled with anxiety their entire life. Others find that their anxiety started later in life. Anxiety can stem from decreased mental capacity due to Alzheimer's disease or other brain problems as well as from an increase in physical ailments and worries.

Discussion

How is depression different from anxiety?

How many of our residents, do you think, deal with one of these diagnoses?

Our nursing team, social services team, and department directors work hard to be sure that residents with depression and/or anxiety are diagnosed and treated appropriately. As members of the activity department, it is important for us to recognize how depression and anxiety can affect participation in leisure pursuits.

Discussion

Can you think of a time recently when a resident did not participate in an activity due to depression or anxiety?

How do you know if a resident is suffering with depression or anxiety? Does that affect your invitations to programs for that person?

If you notice signs and symptoms of depression or anxiety in a resident, whom should you report that information to?

If you have questions about what behaviors are symptoms of depression or anxiety, whom can you ask here at our community to find out more?

Now let's look at how depression and anxiety specifically affect activity programming.

Depression

Depression can cause a resident to isolate. It is awful, because isolation only increases the feelings of sadness and loneliness that come out of depression. A resident who is suffering from depression might decline your invitations to attend programs that he or she once enjoyed. If you notice that a resident is isolating himself or herself, be sure to let nursing and your department director know of the change. We want to be sure that we put residents we are concerned about on our care plan team review. Then everyone keeps a close eye on them, including the doctor. In the meantime, you can choose to treat each of them with a little extra TLC. While it might be easiest to stop asking them to activities because they only decline, continue asking. If you have time, stop in to visit more often. Offer to bring in independent leisure materials that they might enjoy.

Depression can also cause residents to lose confidence or feel unsure of themselves. Residents who are depressed might need a little extra attention and praise from you both during groups and after groups. Praise the residents for attending and for participating. Acknowledge that while it might have been hard for a resident to attend the group, you are glad that he or she did. Consider sitting an unsure resident next to one of your social butterflies in the group, to assure that the resident will feel welcome.

Depression can cause a resident to feel like he or she has nothing to offer. Combat this by asking the resident to help out in some way. Could the resident pass out newspapers, stuff envelopes for marketing, or water and care for the community plants? Giving depressed residents something meaningful to do is an important way to help them feel better.

Discussion

What are some techniques that have helped you get a resident with depression involved?

Are you concerned right now about a particular resident with depression? Let's brainstorm together on ways that we can help meet the needs of this resident.

Anxiety

Anxiety causes people to feel constantly worried or nervous. Imagine a moment in your life when you felt very nervous. Now, imagine that you feel that way all the time. What an awful way to live! We work hard to be sure that residents who live with anxiety have appropriate treatment. However, if you notice that a resident is acting more and more anxious in groups or in your interactions, please be sure to let nursing staff and your department director know. We will investigate and make adjustments to the care plan.

Anxiety can make decision making extremely difficult or even impossible. A resident with anxiety might find choosing whether to attend afternoon exercise an impossible decision. You can gently make the decision for the resident by offering the invitation as a statement and not a question. For example, don't say, "Millie, would you like to come to craft class?" Instead, try saying, "Hi Millie, let's take a walk down to craft class." Millie can always decline to walk with you or leave the craft class once she is there, but this allows Millie to not worry about the initial decision.

Anxiety can cause a resident to be uncomfortable or even frightened in large groups. If a resident seems extra nervous in a large group setting, invite that resident to smaller group programs or one-on-one interactions. Anxiety can also lower tolerance for stimulation. Residents with anxiety might not enjoy a loud group or a multisensory experience such as a performance or social activity. Instead, invite those residents to quieter events so that they feel comfortable and relaxed.

Anxiety can get worse in the evening, especially for those who have Alzheimer's disease or other dementias. You have heard the phrase "sundowner syndrome." In order to decrease anxiety in the evening hours for these residents, consider planning relaxing and low-key programs for this time.

Finally, anxiety can decrease the attention span. A resident living with severe anxiety might not be able to focus on an activity for very long. Plan on keeping things moving along for that resident during the group. If the resident is at a social, ask the resident to help pass out napkins or drinks. Then ask the resident to assist with something else 15-30 minutes later. It will keep the resident engaged and focused on something besides the anxiety.

Discussion

What are some ways that you adapt your program or invitation for someone who has anxiety?

Is there a particular resident with some anxiety-related issues that we can brainstorm about so that we can meet his or her needs better?

Inservice #22
Depression and Anxiety

Inservice Overview: Information about depression and anxiety, and how it might affect participation in programs

Presented by:______________________________

Date:______________________________

Start Time:______________________________

End Time:______________________________

NAME	DEPARTMENT

23.
The Short-Term Resident

Working with short-term residents: expectations and programming.

Topics
Description of the "typical" short-term resident, including their expectations and how to reach them.

Who to Invite
Activity staff, CNA staff who lead activity programs, director of nursing or assistant director of nursing, care plan coordinator, social services staff.

Time
30-40 minutes.

Supplies
Inservice sign-in sheet.
Dry erase board and markers, or just a large piece of paper and markers.

Review Material
Community-specific tools.
State-specific regulatory information.

Content Reminders
Use lots of resident-specific examples and discussion to make this training even more meaningful.

Programming for short-term residents has been an important topic in skilled nursing over the past decade. Health care professionals everywhere want to know about the "typical" short-term resident. Some of the questions include: What do they want? How can we get them to come to our community for their care needs? Should we devote entire wings of our communities for this population? How do we prepare our staff for these residents?

For us in activities, we have noticed an increased need to program for a short-term resident. Activity professionals want to know how to get short-term residents involved in groups, how to encourage them to come out of their room for activities besides therapy, and how to be sure that their leisure needs are being met.

Discussion

What is a short-term resident? Give an example of a current resident who is short term.

Does our community serve a lot of short-term residents?

As we learn more about the typical short-term resident, please keep in mind that no two residents are the same. They do not always share these preferences or expectations. What we are looking for are qualities that many of them share that make them different from residents who stay longer.

Short-term residents are at our community for a short time only, typically no longer than 100 days. These residents are usually younger. They typically have had a medical procedure that requires inpatient therapy after the procedure. These residents receive intensive therapy services, both physical and occupational. They are often in quite a bit of pain upon admission to our community. The typical short-term resident was living at home and plans to return home without any assistance upon discharge. These residents typically see therapy as their main focus while they are here at our community. Getting stronger means they get to go home quicker.

They have strong social support, sometimes a living spouse as well as active family members. Short-term residents are very active in their own plan of care. Although they may involve family members and friends in their decision making, typically these residents make their own decisions.

Short-term residents are typically more technology-savvy and want to stay plugged in. Many will bring in smart phones, laptops, iPads, and/or reading tablets. They typically expect wireless internet access. They also prefer larger, flat-screen televisions with a variety of channel choices.

These residents tend to be health conscious and prefer to have food choices that reflect healthy diets. A short-term resident also typically prefers a light lunch and a heavier dinner. Many communities offer the opposite — a heavier lunch and light dinner. Dining might find that they need to work with these short-term residents on both food choices and meal timing.

Let's take a look at what a typical short-term resident might look like. Mrs. Anderson is 66 and her doctor recommends a knee replacement. She still works part-time as a marketing consultant. She knows that while she could return home after her replacement, a skilled nursing environment will be much more beneficial. Pain control, medical care, and more intensive therapy will be provided on-site. Plus, Mrs. Anderson lives in a two-story townhouse and knows that she will not be able to get up the stairs to her bedroom for at least a few weeks. She does not want her husband to be her primary caregiver, as he works full time. So she chooses to come to a rehabilitation center after a three-night stay in the hospital to fulfill Medicare requirements. Mrs. Anderson does extensive research before her surgery. She calls a few local nursing homes, talks to her friends for recommendations, and tours a few different options. She asks lots of questions regarding therapy services, food choices, wireless internet access, and nursing ratios before making her final decision. Most likely, she sets up her admission date in advance. She might even give the admission coordinator at the nursing home all of her paperwork before she even enters the hospital for her knee replacement. She is planning on staying for about five weeks, but only plans to take off work for three weeks. She will be answering emails and developing marketing plans for her part-time job during the last two weeks of her stay at our community.

Discussion

So far, do these characteristics sound like our short-term residents?

What else could you add that you have noticed to be a shared quality, expectation, situation, or preference for our short-term residents?

Our short-term resident typically comes with a few barriers to getting involved with our programming. The first barrier is a desire by some short-term residents to not be associated with our long-term residents, for a variety of reasons. However, other short-term residents enjoy visiting and caring for our long-term residents. In my experience, it is best to observe the short-term resident to see which of these choices he or she prefers. If a short-term resident enjoys being a part of the lives of our long-term residents, you can get him or her involved with volunteering to do one-on-one visits, helping out with group activities, etc. Best practice in other communities with a large population of short-term residents is to essentially run two separate programming calendars, one for long-term residents and one for short-term residents.

Discussion

What do you think about the two-calendar idea? Would it work here? How would those two calendars look different in regards to programs offered, timing, etc.?

Another programming roadblock that you might see with the short-term resident is a decreased interest in group programs. Short-term residents are typically most interested in therapy sessions. They decline activity invitations because they are waiting on their therapy session, are attending a therapy session, or are too tired from a therapy session.

We must understand and respect the resident's desire for therapy. This resident wants to get home. They know they must get stronger to do that, and therapy is their tool to get stronger. This should not be a frustration for us in activities because our goal — and what is required by federal regulations — is to provide each resident with the activities and amount of activities that he or she wishes to have. One possibility is partnering with therapists for some group programs that are both therapeutic and activities. For example, could we work with therapy and have one or two therapists assist us with leading exercise class or even Wii groups?

Discussion

How do we program for these residents? What barriers do we see?

What are the ethical considerations related to trying to convince short-term residents to be involved in activities?

What kinds of programming might interest residents who are mostly focused on therapy in getting involved in the activities program?

We have to reach our short-term residents differently and we need to adjust our expectations. These residents are typically able to make their own leisure choices. They can usually pursue their interests on their own with little intervention or set-up from us. We must get to know these residents and their interests, and be sure to chart what they are doing during their downtime. Checking their email or reading their Kindle is a leisure pursuit. So is watching their favorite football team or browsing through Facebook. We must have items available to them to help them meet their interests. Current magazines, iPods, handheld electronic games, and even computers or laptops are a good place to start.

Discussion

What do we currently have available for short-term residents who do not want to attend group programs?

What could we do better in terms of offering materials?

Inservice #23
The Short-Term Resident

Inservice Overview: Description of the "typical" short-term resident, including their expectations and how to reach them

Presented by:______________________________

Date:______________________________

Start Time:______________________________

End Time:______________________________

NAME	DEPARTMENT

24.
The Enduring Human Spirit: Sam's Command Performance

An Alzheimer's case study.

Topics
Putting the pieces of the puzzle together — looking at a real-life scenario and finding how we can best serve the resident as an interdisciplinary team.

Who to Invite
Activity staff, CNA staff who lead activity programs, representatives from the interdisciplinary team.

Time
30-40 minutes.

Supplies
Inservice sign-in sheet.
Copies of "A Command Performance," pages 132-135 of *The Enduring Human Spirit* by Charles Tindell. (Idyll Arbor grants the owner of this book permission to make copies of the story and the associated questions for participants in this inservice.)
Dry-erase board (or large piece of paper) and markers.

Content Reminders
We serve our residents best when we work together. The quality of life for our residents is like a puzzle. Each department holds a different piece, a totally unique way of connecting and serving that resident. If we work together and communicate with one another, we can share our knowledge and our gifts to best serve the resident.

Let's put the puzzle of Sam together. First, let's take a moment to read his story. Then we'll work together to answer some questions.

Discussion

What did you think of this story? Did it remind you of any of our residents?

Let's take a moment to complete a mock interdisciplinary team assessment. Let's write down facts that we know about Sam. We should incorporate as many facts as we can so that we can get to know him better — his medical history of dementia, his love of the piano, etc.

What are some ways that we can serve Sam's family? How can we ease their anxiety about moving him to this community? How can we get them involved with his care and his life here?

Let's say that Sam gets agitated and wanders in the evenings. What are five interventions that all staff, no matter the department, can do with Sam to ease his anxiety?

How can dining get involved with Sam's plan of care?

How can we involve volunteers in Sam's life?

How can the maintenance team get involved in Sam's life?

Sam's Command Performance

From *The Enduring Human Spirit* by Charles Tindell

Every week Sam (he prefers to be called Sam rather than Samuel) provides special music by playing the piano for the worship service in one of the wings of our Alzheimer's Care Center. Sam himself is one of the residents in the Center. By his own admission, he isn't a particularly religious person. Yet, by his own choice, he is there every week for the service. He learned the piano as a young man, and regularly played in piano lounges wherever he lived. It wasn't his full-time job but his avocation. Sam loves to play the piano. It is part of who he is.

"Do you think God will like what I play?" Sam asks as he slowly rises from his chair to take his place at the piano. For Sam, it is not a frivolous question.

"Of course, Sam," I reply. "God will enjoy it."

Sam smiles and looks pleased that he is about to play for such a prestigious audience as God. Knowing Sam, he will perform as if he were performing before a packed concert hall; or perhaps a more suitable analogy, he will play as if he were playing in a crowded piano lounge with standing room only. As Sam reaches the piano he pauses, looks at me, and asks, "Are you sure?" As he asks his question, he points upward, surmising I would know whom he was asking about.

"Yes, Sam, I'm sure."

Sam adjusts the piano seat and sits. He stands up again to move the seat ever so slightly, and after he sits again, he lightly fingers the piano keys without producing a sound. After stretching his arms, he announces he is ready. It is a ritual he no doubt acquired over the years. There is no need to adjust any sheet music as part of his ritual since Sam plays from memory. I nod to give him the go ahead, and before I get a chance to sit down, Sam is already pounding out the tune *Alley Cat.* It is one of three tunes he usually plays for God, often times mixing the melodies of all three. Those in attendance, however, do not notice nor seem to care because they are too busy tapping their feet. I can imagine God doing likewise as Sam glances up toward the ceiling every now and then.

We have a sixty-bed Alzheimer's Care Center at our facility. It is divided into three wings or pods as they are sometimes called. Each wing has an all-purpose room referred to as the Great Room. On this morning we are using that room for our worship. Once the service is over, the residents will stay for coffee and cookies served by volunteers. This afternoon the residents will gather in that space for one of their favorite activities — bingo. At other times during the day, the room is used for exercises, watching television, listening to music, reading the paper, or doing jigsaw puzzles. Besides these activities, the room also serves as an area for the residents to pace in and out of throughout the day and, as can be the case of those with Alzheimer's, throughout the night as well.

The wing where, this morning, we are hearing *Alley Cat* is the South Wing, the wing where Sam is a resident. Those who live there are in the middle stages of Alzheimer's. Those who reside in the North Wing are in the advanced stages while those in the West Wing are in its early stages. While those with Alzheimer's can prove to be difficult to handle in any given situation, Sam's friendly smile and engaging personality always has a calming effect upon those who have come for the worship service. He is seen as a nice person who loves to give of himself to others by playing the piano; it is part of who Sam is.

Sam became a resident several years ago after his family reluctantly decided that they could no longer take care of him. Although Sam had physical problems due to the natural process of aging, that was not the determining factor for placement. It was his increasing symptoms of dementia that made the decision necessary. Sam's continual pacing at all hours of the day and night, along with his irregular sleep habits, were draining family members of their energy.

What little energy they had left was quickly used up when he began to wander outside without regard to weather or his own safety. That proved to be the last straw. As one of his family members said, sighing in a voice too tired to care whether she was heard, "The emotional and physical energy … I just … just didn't have any left to worry about his safety."

Placing Sam in the Alzheimer's Care Center was an agonizing decision for the family. It was made only slightly easier because Sam's adjustment to his new home went relatively smoothly and because he was now in a secured environment. With his various aches and pains, Sam realized that, as he said with a laugh at the time of his admission, "I'm not as young as I used to be." Family members noted that it was his way of expressing that he realized that something was changing in his life.

If you were to visit with Sam, you would find him to be a personable man who likes to talk about the traveling he has done in his life. Over the years, Sam traveled all over the world with his work, and continued to travel in his retirement years. Proud of his trips, he has several photo albums of the places he has been. If you expressed even a hint of interest, Sam would get the photograph albums from his dresser drawer to share the pictures of the countries he had visited.

Although he only occasionally remembers where the photographs were taken, he does recognize himself in them, commenting that the picture was taken when he was younger. As for the other people in the photos, including his family, he shakes his head and confesses with a half smile, "I don't know who they are. I guess I don't remember so good anymore." Sam sometimes continues to stare at a particular photograph before turning the page as he tries to remember who those *strangers* are that were standing next to him.

When Sam sits down at the piano to provide the special music for our worship service, I never know what he will play, nor do I always recognize immediately what he does play because of his tendency to blend the tunes. Besides *Alley Cat*, he usually plays *Mexicali Rose,* or *Let Me Call You Sweetheart*, and upon occasion, other mixtures of tunes that neither I nor the music therapist recognize. After he finishes playing, we show our appreciation by applauding. Sam bows, looks upward with raised bushy eyebrows, and with his hand above his head, he points toward the ceiling and bows again.

"Do you think God liked that?" he asked me after he had taken his bows and was shuffling back to his chair to sit with the other residents.

"I know God enjoyed that," I replied.

"That's good," Sam replied, smiling. "I enjoy playing for God."

When Sam plays *Alley Cat*, we use it as a lead-in to talk about cats, dogs, canaries, and any other pets the residents may have had when they were younger. The message I try to get across is that all of these creatures are part of creation, and thus, are reminders of the Creator. We do the same with *Mexicali Rose*, only we talk about the many varieties of flowers within creation, and, as a follow-up, we sing the old-time favorite gospel hymn *In the Garden.* The tune *Let Me Call You Sweetheart* presented a little more of a challenge, but it was decided that this is simply another way of God expressing love for us. All of these connections might raise a few eyebrows among professors and students of theology, but they are meaningful connections and bring smiles of acknowledgment from those in the South Wing of the Alzheimer's Care Center, especially to a piano player by the name of Sam who feels privileged in being the opening act for God. Playing the piano for God is part of who Sam is now.

Questions

1. Sam's family talked about how hard it was to place him in a facility:
   a. What kind of support is offered in your community to families with an elderly person who may need to go into a facility? Are there things that could be done that are not being done now?

   b. What support do the facilities in your area offer? What else could they do? If you are part of a facility, discuss what your plans are to meet the needs of resident families.
   c. Whose "job" is it to offer support to families? What kind of training could be given so that *all* of the people in contact with the elderly and their families are able to give support?

2. Sam had a photo album to share. Discuss benefits of having families putting one together for their loved one. How might the caregivers also benefit from this?

3. Discuss what your community could offer in terms of ongoing educational opportunities for families dealing with Alzheimer's.
   a. Who offers such educational opportunities to your community?
   b. What would be the benefits of offering such programs as 3 and 3a? Who would be responsible for starting such programs?

4. If you do *not* have a music therapist available, in what ways are you using music to help the elderly? What could be done that isn't being done now?

5. What other kind of sensory experiences are you providing for your elderly? e.g., smells, touch, and hearing (familiar sounds such as trains bring back memories).

6. Evaluate living quarters for Alzheimer's: Would you put your loved one there? Why or why not? What would you suggest to improve it? (If you're not sure, ask the families who have relatives in an Alzheimer's unit).

7. Discuss the pros and cons of the following question: Should Alzheimer's residents be housed according to what stage of the disease they are in?

If this story and questions has helped you and others learn more about care for our elders, please consider reading and discussing some of the other 43 lessons in *The Enduring Human Spirit: Thought-Provoking Stories on Caring for Our Elders* by Charles Tindell. Available through your favorite bookstore.

Inservice #24

The Enduring Human Spirit: Sam's Command Performance

Inservice Overview: Putting the pieces of the puzzle together — looking at a real life scenario and finding how we can best serve the resident as an interdisciplinary team

Presented by:________________________________

Date:________________________________

Start Time:________________________________

End Time:________________________________

NAME	DEPARTMENT

25.
The Enduring Human Spirit: Alfred's Friends for Life

A case study of wellness, behavior prevention, and de-escalation.

Topics
A case study to determine dimensions of wellness, leisure's role in prevention of negative behaviors, and de-escalation.

Who to Invite
Activity staff, CNA staff, interdisciplinary team staff.

Time
30-40 minutes.

Supplies
Inservice sign-in sheet.
Copies of "Friends for Life," pages 50-55 of *The Enduring Human Spirit* by Charles Tindell. (Idyll Arbor grants the owner of this book permission to make copies of the story and the associated questions for participants in this inservice.)
Dry-erase board (or large piece of paper) and markers to brainstorm ideas or write down action items.

Content Reminders
Leisure plays an important role in preventing resident behaviors and de-escalating those behaviors. But, everyone must know what approaches work, not just the activity staff. Also, we must work together to find out what is causing the behaviors in the first place.

Let's read the story of Alfred together and see how the dimensions of wellness played a part in his behaviors. First, let's take a moment to read his story. Then we'll work together to answer some questions.

Discussion

What did you think of this story? Did it remind you of any of our residents?

In Alfred's story, what dimension of wellness was not being met and that ultimately caused his wandering/agitation? (social)

What was he seeking when he left his unit?

As the CNAs were trying to get Alfred to return to the unit, what approaches were they using? Was it working?

What approach did the Chaplain use to redirect Alfred and calm his agitation? Did it work?

How was the Chaplain able to meet Alfred's social dimension of wellness? What was the result?

If Alfred begins to seem agitated or show signs of wandering in the future, what could staff do to ease his agitation?

What approaches or activities could be built into Alfred's care plan so that the agitation and wandering behaviors are prevented altogether?

Friends for Life

From *The Enduring Human Spirit* by Charles Tindell

"Aghhh … Let … me … aghhhh … go," Alfred screamed as if his very life was being threatened. "You're … not … me … back … aghhhh!"

Even though Alfred was nearly slipping out of his wheelchair, he continued to hang on to the edge of the hallway door with a strength well belying his eighty-five years. With one hand clutching the door handle and the other having a firm grip on the edge of the door itself, he was prepared to make his stand. He was determined not to go back. Not now. Not after he had come this far.

Two nursing aides had been sent to bring Alfred back to the third floor of the Chronic Care Center where he was a resident. The aides had caught up with him in "the ramp," a first floor hallway that connects the Chronic Care Center to another part of the facility that houses the Assisted Living apartments, the Chapel, and what is known as Town Square.

Halfway down the ramp where Alfred was at the moment are two fire doors, doors that automatically close whenever the fire alarm sounds. It was one of these fire doors that he had latched onto, tenaciously refusing to let go. The aides tried to persuade him to return to his room but were not being very successful. Alfred was becoming more belligerent by the moment; the aides, more desperate.

"Alfred, you've got to come back, please," pleaded one of the aides, looking to his partner for help.

"Aghhh … no … nooo!" Alfred cried, looking at them as if they were the enemy; in his mind, they no doubt were.

Since neither of the aides had the time to spend escorting Alfred wherever he had decided and was determined to go, they didn't relish the unpleasant task that lay before them. They looked at one another and nodded their heads knowingly; both knew that it was a difficult situation as they talked quietly between themselves about what their next move should be.

I heard the yelling from my office and went to investigate. When I came upon the scene, Alfred was still hanging on to the door and the two aides were still trying to prevail upon him to return to his floor. As I was later told, one of the aides had initially attempted to turn Alfred's wheelchair around. This action prompted his yelling and grabbing hold of the door. The aide, startled by the outburst, quickly let go of his wheelchair. From that point on, if either of the aides got too close, Alfred wildly kicked out at them. He wouldn't listen to their explanation that they were responsible for him and they needed to bring him back.

Alfred, as he later told me his side of the story, had managed to get down to the first floor by sneaking onto the elevator. He had wheeled up to the elevator doors where he lived on the third floor and just waited. He didn't have to wait long before the doors opened, letting some visitors off. When the visitors got off, Alfred wheeled on. Once he was on, he figured he was home free.

As soon as Alfred got on the elevator, however, the staff were alerted immediately when an alarm sounded at the nurses' station. A device called a Wanderguard that Alfred wore on his wrist had activated the alarm; it is an electronic wristband that many residents wear. When Alfred got on the elevator, a circuit box located on the wall by the elevator doors picked up the signals from his electronic wristband. Once the signals are detected, it activates an alarm at the nurses' station that buzzes quite loudly. The wristband is for resident safety. Those residents, like Alfred, who are apt to wander without regard for their own well-being, wear it. The danger is that residents may not only leave the floors where their rooms are, but also, if given the opportunity, the facility itself.

Being in a wheelchair is not a deterrent to a resident who is determined to leave the building. One day, as I was leaving work, I came upon a resident in his wheelchair who was outside in a temperature of thirty degrees. This man wore slippers but had no socks on and was dressed in slacks and a short-sleeved shirt. Although shivering and complaining about being a little cold, he was still headed away from the building toward a busy main road.

He was disoriented and sufficiently confused not to have been able to return to the building himself. He wasn't wearing an electronic wristband and, as we now know in hindsight, should have been. The very next day this man received a Wanderguard. I was reminded of him as I was dealing with Alfred now.

"What's going on, Alfred?" I asked in a light-hearted tone while signaling to the aides that I would stay with him and they could go.

Both aides were grateful and looked relieved as they said their good-byes to Alfred while informing me they needed to go back and attend to their other duties. Having thanked them for their concern about Alfred, I assured them that I'd see to it that he would be brought back to the third floor.

"See you up on third, Alfred," one of the aides said as he looked back and waved; the other aide simply smiled and waved. It was obvious that they cared about him even after having gone through such a trying experience.

"Not … aghhh … going … good-bye," Alfred yelled. "I … aghhh … good-bye … see … you." He didn't wave but hung on to the door until the two of them were gone. It was only after the aides turned the corner of the hallway and were out of sight that Alfred loosened his grip.

"Shall we go for a little ride?" I asked. After he nodded yes, I began to slowly push his wheelchair in the direction he had been originally headed.

"They … he … go … aghhh … damn … not … nurse … room … I …" Alfred's response still showed a great deal of agitation. The agitation, I suspected, was a combination of his being upset about what had just taken place as well as a high level of frustration on his part from not being able to verbally express himself the way he wanted. If he could have expressed himself, perhaps none of this would have happened.

Alfred had had a mild stroke two months earlier that affected his speech. His stroke, along with increasing signs of memory loss and resulting confusion, had precipitated his move to the Chronic Care Center. The move had been difficult for him because he had left friends behind in the Board and Care building where he had lived for over two years. He was determined to return to his previous living area, and had worked very hard with the speech therapists. Through weeks of therapy he learned to communicate. By concentrating and speaking slowly, Alfred could verbalize his thoughts; what came out might be a little choppy, but was reasonably understandable. Unfortunately, his sentences would become garbled and disjointed whenever he became agitated.

"Do you want to go down to the coffee shop and see who's there?" I asked. "Perhaps we could look around at some of the stuff being sold, and we might even run into someone you know. Wouldn't that be nice?"

"Yes … ah … yes," Alfred replied, nodding his head in agreement. He was calmer now, knowing that he wasn't going to be taken back to his room.

When Alfred and I got to the area outside the coffee shop (an area called the Promenade), we discovered that it was being used to host the "birthday of the month" party for those residents who lived in Assisted Living and Board and Care. Tables had been set up, and cake and ice cream were being served. There were close to a hundred residents in attendance; they had come to celebrate the birthdays of a dozen or so of their peers.

Alfred's friends and former neighbors immediately recognized him. As I wheeled him around, going from table to table, many greeted him with a warm smile and a hearty handshake.

"Hi, there, Alfred," a petite, silver-haired, attractive woman called out in a friendly voice; it was Mabel, one of his good friends.

"Nice to see you, Alfred," another said.

"We miss you," Milton exclaimed as he wheeled his wheelchair up to Alfred. "When are you coming back? Soon I hope."

"Oh, look," Bob exclaimed to the group at his table, "there's Alfred." He, along with the others at the table, raised their cups of coffee in a toast.

Alvin hollered and waved at Alfred from across the way, offering him a welcoming smile. "You're looking great, my friend."

Besides the verbal greetings, there were handshakes, pats on the back, and even a few hugs. The effect upon Alfred was amazing as he smiled and laughed; all signs of agitation were gone.

Although his sentences were still a little garbled, his friends were able to understand him. Any confusion now was only because of his excitement at seeing his old friends.

After Alfred and I had spent time visiting with his friends, we went into the coffee shop to browse in the general store. After some time passed, I knew I needed to return to the work I had been doing before getting involved with Alfred.

"Alfred, are you ready to head back home?" I asked.

"Uh huh," he replied.

All the way back Alfred and I talked about how gratifying it was for him to see his friends. I told him that he had so many people who cared about him. To each of my comments, Alfred would smile and say, "Uh huh, yes." When I wheeled him past the spot where he had, just a short while ago, hung on so desperately to the door and fought with the two aides, I wondered if it would trigger something within him that would cause him to balk at going back to the third floor. We went past the two fire doors, however, without any indication from Alfred that that had been the spot where he had made his stand.

"It's been a great time," I said to Alfred as I pushed the button for the elevator that would take us back to the third floor. He nodded his head in agreement. We both knew that he had set out to see his friends, and he did it. He was content.

Alfred never returned to live in Board and Care but every so often, the alarm buzzes at the nurses' station on the third floor of the Chronic Care Center. When it does, I suspect it might be Alfred on his way to see his friends again.

Questions

1. Due to Alfred's declining condition, it was necessary to transfer him from one part of the facility to another. What should be required in the policies and procedures for transfers within a facility? What should be done for the resident to make the transition easier?

2. Thinking of the elderly you know:
   a. Is it important to make sure that every elderly person is able to get away from where he or she lives for a change of scenery? Would that enhance the quality of life for the person?
   b. Should facilities have a policy that requires making sure that residents can go to other parts of the facility and other parts of the community?
   c. If your answer is yes to 2b, the issue often raised is "We don't have enough staff time." If, however, you think it is important for the elderly to have a change of scenery from time to time, how could this be accomplished?

3. The aides and Alfred were in engaged in a situation that called for conflict resolution. How would *you* have handled the situation? Is there conflict-resolution training for caretakers and families of the elderly (not only as they deal with the elderly, but also as they deal with one another)? For that matter, should the elderly be taking conflict-resolution training themselves? Discuss why it would be helpful to receive it.

If this story and questions has helped you and others learn more about care for our elders, please consider reading and discussing some of the other 43 lessons in *The Enduring Human Spirit: Thought-Provoking Stories on Caring for Our Elders* by Charles Tindell. Available through your favorite bookstore.

Inservice #25

The Enduring Human Spirit: Alfred's Friends for Life

Inservice Overview: Looking at a case study to determine dimensions of wellness, leisure's role in behavior prevention, and de-escalation

Presented by:____________________

Date:____________________

Start Time:____________________

End Time:____________________

NAME	DEPARTMENT

26.
Nontraditional Inservice Ideas

Ways to transmit information to staff without being in a meeting setting.

When you plan your inservice topics for the month or for the year, consider that not everyone learns best in classroom settings. You might also have a month or months when getting everyone together for a 30-minute inservice seems impossible, for example, during the holiday season or the state survey window.

Here is a list of fun inservices that are based on self-directed learning. Simply pick one to focus on, pass out the supplies to each staff member, give them a deadline for completing the materials, and then have staff sign the inservice sheet when they turn in the completed materials to you. Be sure to be specific about the learning goals on the inservice sign-in sheet so that it is clear what the point was in regards to learning.

Find an article in a magazine, journal, or even a professional newsletter, such as *Creative Forecasting,* that addresses a topic of interest. Pass out a copy of the article as well as a few questions based on the article to each staff member. Have staff read the article during down time at work — not during their lunch or break time, it must be during paid time — and then turn in the answers to the questions to you. Include the article and answers to the questions with the inservice sheet when you turn it in to the HR department for filing.

Create a scavenger hunt. Identify and list 10 things in your community. Pass out the list to each staff member and give a timeframe to find the items. The staff person writes the locations of the items and returns the completed paper to you. Pick items that you want them to use more often or be more familiar with. Ideas might include: where do we keep the sensory kits, where does Mrs. Smith keep her knitting needles, where is Mr. Villagio's family photo album, etc. Include the completed forms with the inservice sheet when you turn them in for filing.

Create a job-shadowing opportunity. Pass out a sheet to each staff member with a few questions that they need to ask another staff member. For example, ask a CNA what the hardest part of her job is, ask a dining team member when they are busiest during their shift, etc. This will allow for staff to get to know the staff in other departments and gain respect for different jobs throughout the community. Turn in the completed sheets with the inservice form.

Create a "Name That Resident" handout. Questions are based on unique residents' histories and might include: which of our residents fought in WWII, how many residents on the second floor speak another language, etc. Each staff member completes the handout and returns it to you.

Have each staff member sign up to attend a stand-up meeting or a care plan meeting with you. After they attend, the person writes a paragraph or two describing the experience and what was learned from attending the meeting. Attach the paragraphs to the inservice sheet.

Have staff members sign up for a time to watch you to lead an activity. Ideally, staff would pick an activity that they do not feel confident leading or one where they would like extra tips. Once you lead the group, they write a paragraph or two about what they learned from watching you lead the group and then give it to you.

Inservice #26

Inservice Topic

Inservice Overview: Using nontraditional ways to learn about residents and our community.

Presented by: Self-directed learning

Date:

Start Time:

End Time:

NAME	DEPARTMENT

About the Author

Haley Burress has a Master's Degree in Recreation Therapy and 15 years of experience working with seniors in all levels of care including independent living, assisted living, skilled nursing facility care, memory care, and adult day services. Haley has been at a director level or higher throughout her career and has managed teams of up to 60 people.

Haley consults and speaks on a variety of topics including programming ideas, strategies for improving resident care, and how to make the activity director job as easy and fun as possible. She currently writes for caregivers — professionals and family members — fulltime, including *52 Weeks Studying the Word* — a Bible study resource for seniors, content for ActivityDirector.com, Activity Connection, Companion Radio, LotsaHelpingHands and others. She specializes in giving her readers reliable information that will leave them feeling empowered and inspired.

In her spare time, you can find Haley playing superheroes with her son Jackson or hiking with her husband Derrick. She loves running, exploring the outdoors, and brownies — not necessarily all at once.

CPSIA information can be obtained
at www.ICGtesting.com
Printed in the USA
FSOW03n2242061216
28021FS

9 781611 580426